Springer Series on Child and Family Studies

Series Editor
Nirbhay N. Singh
Medical College of Georgia
Augusta University
Augusta, GA, USA

The *Springer Series on Child and Family Studies* addresses fundamental psychological, educational, social, and related issues within the context of child and family research. Volumes published in this series examine clinical topics with an additional focus on epidemiological, developmental, and life span issues. Leading scholars explore such factors as race and immigration, parenting, and the effects of war and violence on military families and unite a vast literature into a comprehensive series of related research volumes.

More information about this series at http://www.springer.com/series/13095

Keith C Radley • Evan H. Dart

Social Skills Teaching for Individuals with Autism

Integrating Research into Practice

Springer

Keith C Radley
Department of Educational Psychology
University of Utah
Salt Lake City, UT, USA

Evan H. Dart
Department of Educational and Psychological Studies
University of South Florida
Tampa, FL, USA

ISSN 2570-0421 ISSN 2570-043X (electronic)
Springer Series on Child and Family Studies
ISBN 978-3-030-91664-0 ISBN 978-3-030-91665-7 (eBook)
https://doi.org/10.1007/978-3-030-91665-7

This Springer imprint is published by the registered company Springer Nature Switzerland AG
The registered company address is: Gewerbestrasse 11, 6330 Cham, Switzerland

To D.T. and family

Acknowledgments

The authors would like to thank Katrina Scarimbolo and Paige Dubrow for their assistance in formatting chapters and references in preparation for publication.

Contents

About the Authors

Keith C Radley is an associate professor in the Department of Educational Psychology at the University of Utah. He completed his doctoral training in educational psychology at the University of Utah in 2011. Dr. Radley is a licensed psychologist, board-certified behavior analyst, and nationally certified school psychologist. His research interests include social skills teaching and other supports for individuals with developmental disabilities, student behavior support in educational settings, and data collection, visualization, and analysis within single case design.

Evan H. Dart is an associate professor in the Department of Educational and Psychological Studies at the University of South Florida. He graduated from the school psychology doctoral program at Louisiana State University in 2013. Dr. Dart is a licensed psychologist and a board-certified behavior analyst whose research interests include school-based interventions for students at-risk for behavioral disorders, behavior assessment methods, and the use of progress monitoring data to make decisions about student performance.

Chapter 1
Autism Spectrum Disorder

In what has become a seminal article in the field of clinical psychiatry, Leo Kanner (1943) described 11 cases of children with "infantile autism." Kanner described the children as lacking social instincts, atypical use of language, and insistence on sameness and consistency. Independently and simultaneously, Hans Asperger (1944) also described children who demonstrated social isolation, atypical verbal and nonverbal communication skills, and a restricted and narrow focus on interests—though several differences were noted (e.g., good cognitive and linguistic skills observed in Asperger's sample). Both Kanner and Asperger used the term "autism" to describe the observed cluster of behaviors—a term previously utilized by Eugen Bleuler to describe symptoms of schizophrenia. Although the characteristics described by Kanner and Asperger have corresponded with several different diagnostic classifications since Infantile Autism first appeared in the Diagnostic and Statistical Manual, 3rd Edition (1980), they currently correspond with the Diagnostic and Statistical Manual, 5th Edition's (DSM-5; American Psychiatric Association, 2013) criteria for autism spectrum disorder (ASD).

Classification Criteria

As described in the DSM-5, ASD is defined by five diagnostic criteria. First, there must be persistent deficits in social communication and social interaction. These deficits must be apparent across a variety of contexts, such as school, home, and community settings. Three primary areas are considered as part of deficits in social communication and social interaction: (1) deficits in social-emotional reciprocity, or the ability to initiate, respond to, and maintain give-and-take of social interactions; (2) deficits in use or integration of nonverbal communication, as evidenced by features such as atypicalities in use and modulation of eye contact, facial

K. C Radley, E. H. Dart, *Social Skills Teaching for Individuals with Autism*,
Springer Series on Child and Family Studies,
https://doi.org/10.1007/978-3-030-91665-7_1

expressions, and body language; and (3) deficits in establishing, maintaining, and understanding relationships. Although deficits in language skills are not required as part of the DSM-5 diagnostic criteria, they may have a substantial impact on an individual's ability to engage in meaningful social communication and interaction.

The second diagnostic criterion requires the presence of restricted and repetitive patterns of behavior, interests, or activities. For this criterion, an individual must display at least two of the following: stereotyped or repetitive speech (e.g., repetition of phrases), stereotyped interaction with and use of objects (e.g., lining up toys), or repetitive motor behaviors; insistence on sameness, inflexibility with respect to routines, or ritualized patterns of behavior (e.g., rituals for getting dressed, greeting others); restricted, fixated interests that are atypical in focus or intensity; and hypo- or hyper-reactivity to sensory stimulation or an atypical interest in sensory elements of one's environment (e.g., smelling objects). Although both the DSM-5 and IDEA describe impairments in social communication and restricted and repetitive behaviors separately, these two features are often inextricably intertwined. For example, an individual with ASD may seek to initiate conversations about a particular topic that involves a restricted interest without participating in social give-and-take whereby the topic may shift between the interests of two or more parties or settle on a shared interest.

Third, the aforementioned characteristics must be observed during the early developmental period; however, the DSM-5 specifies that they might not be observed until social demands on the individual are increased (e.g., upon school entry) or may be masked by learned compensatory strategies. Fourth and fifth, the characteristics must cause clinically significant impairment in important areas of functioning (e.g., school, vocational, or social settings) and must not better be accounted for by other developmental disabilities (e.g., intellectual disability, global developmental delay), respectively.

Symptom severity is subsequently classified as Level 1 (i.e., "requiring support"), Level 2 ("requiring substantial support"), or Level 3 (i.e., "requiring very substantial support"). This method of classification of symptom severity, a feature introduced with the DSM-5, underscores the nature of a spectrum of autism. Thus, although all individuals who meet diagnostic criteria will present with impacted social communication and restricted, repetitive behaviors, all individuals will demonstrate variations in presentation and support required—ranging from a high degree of independence with some examples of atypical or unsuccessful social interactions to impairments that substantially limit the functional independence of an individual (e.g., severe verbal and nonverbal communication deficits).

Although the diagnostic criteria described in the DSM-5 and other medical classification manuals like it (e.g., International Classification for Diseases, 11th revision; ICD-11; World Health Organization, 2019) are widely utilized in clinical settings, other criteria for identifying individuals with ASD exist. Most notably, the Individuals with Disabilities Improvement Act (IDEIA; 2004) describes criteria for a student to receive a special education classification of Autism within the United States' public education system. Special education classifications provide students with Individualized Education Program (IEPs) which mandate the provision of intensive academic support and other related services (e.g., speech or occupational therapy) based on the unique needs of the student. Section 300.8 (c) (1) of IDEIA defines Autism as a developmental disability, generally evident before age 3, that is often associated with engagement in repetitive activities, resistance to change, and unusual response to sensory stimulation, that adversely impacts educational performance; and is not considered if educational performance is impacted due to emotional disturbance. Specific eligibility criteria vary across states (Pennington et al., 2014), but generally describe that Autism has an adverse educational impact on the student, that the student requires special education services, that Autism is the primary disability, and that significant impairments in verbal and/or nonverbal communication (e.g., lack of and difficulty with social interaction, failure to develop peer relationships).

Although DSM-5 criteria and IDEIA's special education definition have substantial overlap, the additional requirement that students demonstrate a need for special education services may potentially result in individuals receiving a diagnosis of ASD but not being eligible for special education services under the classification of Autism. It is important to note that a medical diagnosis of ASD by a licensed health service professional (e.g., medical doctor, psychologist, psychiatrist) does not guarantee a special education classification of Autism through IDEIA. In fact, the special education evaluation process is most often conducted entirely within the public school system by relevant school staff members (e.g., school psychologists, social workers, special education teachers) with little or no input from outside professionals.

Etiology

The exact etiology of ASD is unclear and it is believed to stem from a combination of genetic and environmental influences; however, research is mixed regarding the extent to whether genetic or environmental factors best explain the development of ASD. For example, Taylor et al. (2020) conducted a study of over 22,000 twin pairs and determined that genetic factors played a more important role than environmental factors in the development of ASD and that this relationship was consistent over the nearly 40 year range covered. On the other hand, Frazier et al. (2014) identified symptom extremity (measured using the Social Responsiveness Scale) as a potentially important variable, with genetic factors becoming more important when ASD symptoms were extreme (i.e., standardized *T* score greater than 70) and less so when symptoms were moderate to mild (i.e., *T* score of 70 or below). Finally, Sealey and colleagues (2015) conducted a comprehensive review of ASD environmental determinants of ASD, concluding that fetal exposure to a variety of chemicals (e.g., fragrances from perfumes, herbicides) may play a role, particularly during early gestation (i.e., 4–18 weeks). Although these studies are just a very small selection of the available evidence, they highlight the complex and varied etiology of ASD;

however, it is clear that no single genetic or environmental factor is solely responsible for its development.

One environmental factor that has received considerable attention in both the scientific community and popular culture as a potential cause of ASD is vaccination. In a now retracted 1998 report published in *The Lancet,* Andrew Wakefield described a link between receipt of the MMR vaccine and development of autism, driving fear among the general public about vaccinations. This fear resulted in a decline in vaccination rates among some developed countries, leading scientists to express concern about the return of preventable diseases (e.g., Pandolfi et al., 2018). The scientific evidence against the proposed link between the MMR vaccine and autism has been accumulating. Recently, Taylor et al. (2014) conducted a meta-analysis of ten studies including over one million participants and concluded that vaccinated individuals were no more likely to develop ASD than those who were not (OR = 0.91; 95% CI = 0.68–1.20). These results provide very convincing evidence that those who receive regular vaccinations are no more likely to develop ASD than those who do not.

Prevalence

Discussion of ASD's etiology often goes hand-in-hand with discussions of its prevalence, which has changed substantially since initial epidemiological studies. In one of the earliest epidemiological studies conducted in the USA, Treffert—using criteria proposed by Kanner—found a prevalence of 0.07 per 10,000. Research in other countries (e.g., Denmark, Japan, United Kingdom) found prevalence rates to be slightly higher; however, rates were generally found to be below 5 per 10,000. Subsequent epidemiological research found an increasing trend in prevalence, with rates increasing to more than 30 cases per 10,000 children in the 1990s (Blaxill, 2004). Since that time, the United States Centers for Disease Control (CDC) has completed surveillance studies. Since the first year of surveillance, the CDC has reported that prevalence has increased from 67 cases per 10,000 children in 2000 to 185 cases per 10,000 children in 2016.

Data presented in many epidemiological studies has primarily focused on clinical diagnosis of ASD. However, studies evaluating special education classification trends have produced similar findings. For example, 93,000 students had an eligibility category of Autism in 93,000—representing 1.53% of all students receiving special education services (Cardinal et al., 2021). In 2015, the number of students with an eligibility category of Autism increased to 538,000, or 8.89% of all students receiving special education services. This nearly sixfold increase is particularly noteworthy, given the relatively unchanged total number of students receiving special education services (Cardinal et al., 2021).

Several factors are likely associated with rising prevalence numbers in both clinical and educational settings. Matson and Kozlowski (2011) identified six factors related to increasing prevalence of ASD. First, and perhaps most frequently noted, are changes in diagnostic criteria over time. Initial estimates by Treffert (1970) were made using criteria proposed by Kanner, with the majority of subsequent epidemiological studies utilizing criteria from the DSM-III (APA, 1980), DSM-IV (APA, 1994), DSM-IV-TR (APA, 2000), and the DSM-5 (APA, 2013). Across each successive version of the DSM, diagnostic criteria were revised and changed, with many suggesting changes have broadened diagnostic criteria (e.g., Lenoir et al., 2009; Wing & Potter, 2002). In one example, King and Bearman (2009) suggested that over 25% of cases in California could be accounted for by changes in diagnostic criteria. In addition to changes in diagnostic criteria, Matson and Kozlowski also identified inaccurate diagnosis, differences in research methodology, environmental factors (e.g., increased survival rates of premature infants), cultural factors, and increased awareness of ASD as contributors to increase in prevalence.

Regarding special education prevalence, the increase in the number of students receiving special education services under the category of Autism without an overall increase in the number of students receiving special education services may be considered in terms of diagnostic substitution. In the case of special education data, specific learning disability classifications have steadily decreased as Autism classifications have increased (Cardinal et al., 2021). Cardinal and colleagues interpret these data as suggesting that individuals with ASD were always present in schools, but that comfort and familiarity of IEP team members with the criteria for Autism, as well as broader awareness of ASD and the availability of resources, have resulted in a degree of diagnostic substitution.

Developmental Trajectories and Outcomes

In considering developmental trajectories and outcomes of individuals with autism spectrum disorder, it is critical to do so with a consideration of the wide variations of presentation that occur due to the spectrum of impact inherent to autism spectrum disorder. As such, developmental trajectories and outcomes may be considered generally, but are unlikely to represent any one particular individual with ASD.

Proximal

Proximal outcomes for children and adolescents with ASD may be considered in a variety of ways, including academic, social outcomes, and mental and behavioral health outcomes. Regarding academic performance, several researchers have found that many children demonstrate variability in achievement—excelling in some areas while struggling in others (e.g., Estes et al., 2011; Jones et al., 2009). For the subset of children who demonstrate academic deficits, factors such as the presence of speech before age 5 and overall language level have been found to be associated with academic performance (e.g., Venter et al., 1992). Although children and adolescents with ASD may present with varying degrees of academic strengths and deficits, academic skills have been found to generally be commensurate with cognitive levels—with children with higher cognitive skills at age 3 and 9 demonstrating greater academic achievement throughout the remainder of their schooling (Kim et al., 2018). Some intervention strategies, such as parent-mediated early intervention, have been found to confer short-term proximal benefit in both cognitive and academic areas (e.g., Green et al., 2010; Kasari et al., 2014).

Similar to academic outcomes, proximal social outcomes have been found to vary substantially across individuals. In general, researchers have found that individuals with fewer deficits tend to have better social outcomes (e.g., Cederland et al., 2008). In general, however, children with ASD have been found to have fewer reciprocal friendships than their typically developing peers (Bauminger et al., 2010), have poorer quality friendships (Calder et al., 2013), are more likely to be isolated during unstructured periods (e.g., recess; Corbett et al., 2014) and experience peer neglect or rejection (Locke et al., 2013). Similar to academic skills, intervention targeting social outcomes has been found to be beneficial in improving short-term outcomes (e.g., Bellini et al., 2007).

ASD symptomatology has also been found to be related to short-term mental and behavioral health outcomes. For example, Salazar et al. (2015) and Moseley and colleagues (2011) found comorbid mental and behavioral health concerns to be present in between 42 and 90% of young children diagnosed with ASD. Even when controlling for factors such as cognitive functioning and emotional/behavioral functioning, researchers have found children with ASD to demonstrate greater likelihood of developing emotional and behavioral problems during early childhood (Saito et al., 2017; Totsika et al., 2011). Similar to the domains previously described, intervention has been found to impact outcomes such as disruptive behavior and hyperactivity (Tarver et al., 2019).

Distal

Research suggests that increasing numbers of individuals with ASD consider post-secondary education as an option following high school (Volkmar et al., 2017). Research by Newman et al. (2011) indicates that approximately 44% of individuals with ASD transitioning from secondary schools enroll in post-secondary education. Despite a substantial proportion of individuals entering post-secondary education, they are at increased risk of leaving prior to completion of a degree (Drake, 2014). For individuals with ASD, post-secondary education is related to greater rates of employment, greater wages, and increased number of hours worked (Whittenburg et al., 2019). Overall, however, individuals with ASD have been found to experience greater rates of unemployment than typically developing peers (Sanford et al., 2011), and most research suggests the majority of adults with ASD experience poor to very poor outcomes related to employment and functional independence (Henninger & Taylor, 2013).

Social outcomes have also been documented to be poor for adults with ASD. Howlin et al. (2013) found that although symptoms of ASD tend to decrease over time, social outcomes were found to be poorer than in childhood. Similar to childhood, adults with ASD often report greater social isolation (Orsmond et al., 2004; Whitehouse et al., 2009), with friendships being less close than their typically developing peers (Baron-Cohen & Wheelwright, 2003). Individuals also have been found to participate in fewer social events and recreational activities (Eaves & Ho, 2008; Howlin et al., 2000). When compared to individuals who received special education services under the categories of intellectual disability, emotional/behavioral disability, or learning disability, adults with ASD were still found to be significantly more isolated and removed from peer interaction (Orsmond et al., 2013). For individuals with higher cognitive and adaptive skills and better conversational skills, social outcomes have been found to be predictive of greater social participation (Farley et al., 2009; Orsmond et al., 2013).

With respect to mental and behavioral health, adults with ASD have been found to continue to demonstrate high rates of comorbid mental and behavioral health concerns (e.g., Croen et al., 2015). Of the comorbid conditions identified, anxiety and depression have been found to occur at particularly high rates (Croen et al., 2015; Lever & Geurts, 2016). Adaptive functioning has been found to be related to increased risk of severe mental and behavioral health concerns (Kraper et al., 2017), with a greater discrepancy between cognitive and adaptive functioning being associated with increased report of depression and anxiety. Similar to children and adolescents with ASD, adults with ASD report substantial rates of bullying—further increasing risk for anxiety (Weiss et al., 2015). Recent research also suggests that individuals with ASD are at increased risk of suicidality and substance use disorders (e.g., Butwicka et al., 2017; Richa et al., 2014).

Conclusion

Over the relatively short period in which ASD has been described and researched, it has gone from being considered a rare condition to one that is frequently identified in school and community settings. Although diagnostic criteria have generally been considered to widen since its first description in the DSM-III, hallmark features of social impairments and restricted and repetitive patterns of behavior have been consistent throughout. Relatedly, intervention supports in ASD frequently target these areas, with social skills teaching being identified as the most frequently implemented intervention in school-based settings (Hess et al., 2008). The remainder of this text will focus first on providing an operational definition of social skills that may be used by practitioners, followed by description of evidence-based social skills teaching strategies that may be considered by interventionists.

References

American Psychiatric Association (APA). (1980). *Diagnostic and statistical manual of mental disorders* (3rd ed.).

American Psychiatric Association (APA). (1994). *Diagnostic and statistical manual of mental disorders* (4th ed.).

American Psychiatric Association (APA). (2000). *Diagnostic and statistical manual of mental disorders* (4th ed., text rev.).

American Psychiatric Association (APA). (2013). *Diagnostic and statistical manual of mental disorders* (5th ed.).

Asperger, H. (1944). Die 'Autistischen Psychopathen' im Kindesalter. *Archivfur Psychiatrie und Nervenkrankheiten, 117*, 76–13.

Baron-Cohen, S., & Wheelwright, S. (2003). The Friendship Questionnaire: An investigation of adults with Asperger syndrome or high-functioning autism, and normal sex differences. *Journal of Autism and Developmental Disorders, 33*, 509–517.

Bauminger, N., Solomon, M., & Rogers, S. J. (2010). Predicting friendship quality in autism spectrum disorders and typical development. *Journal of Autism and Developmental Disorders, 40*, 751–761.

Bellini, S., Peters, J. K., Benner, L., & Hopf, A. (2007). A meta-analysis of school-based social skills interventions for children with autism spectrum disorders. *Remedial and Special Education, 28*, 153–162.

Blaxill, M. F. (2004). What's going on? The question of time trends in autism. *Public Health Reports, 119*, 536–551.

Butwicka, A., Långström, N., Larsson, H., Lundström, S., Serlachius, E., Almqvist, C., et al. (2017). Increased risk for substance use-related problems in autism spectrum disorders: A population-based cohort study. *Journal of Autism and Developmental Disorders, 47*, 80–89.

Calder, L., Hill, V., & Pellicano, E. (2013). 'Sometimes I want to play by myself': Understanding what friendship means to children with autism in mainstream primary schools. *Autism, 17*, 296–316.

Cardinal, D. N., Griffiths, A. J., Maupin, Z. D., & Fraumeni-McBride, J. (2021). An investigation of increased rates of autism in US public schools. *Psychology in the Schools, 58*, 124–140.

Cederland, M., Hagberg, B., Billstedt, E., Gillberg, I., & Gillberg, C. (2008). Asperger syndrome and autism: A comparative longitudinal follow-up study more than 5 years after original diagnosis. *Journal of Autism and Developmental Disorders, 38*, 72–85.

Corbett, B. A., Qualls, L. R., Valencia, B., Fecteau, S. M., & Swain, D. M. (2014). Peer-mediated theatrical engagement for improving reciprocal social interaction in autism spectrum disorder. *Frontiers in Pediatrics, 2*, 1–9.

Croen, L. A., Zerbo, O., Qian, Y., Massolo, M. L., Rich, S., Sidney, S., & Kripke, C. (2015). The health status of adults on the autism spectrum. *Autism, 19*, 814–823.

Drake, S. (2014). College experience of academically successful students with autism. *Journal of Autism, 1*, 1–4.

Eaves, L. C., & Ho, H. H. (2008). Young adult outcome of autism spectrum disorders. *Journal of Autism and Developmental Disorders, 38*, 739–747.

Estes, A., Rivera, V., Bryan, M., Cali, P., & Dawson, G. (2011). Discrepancies between academic achievement and intellectual ability in higher-functioning school-aged children with autism spectrum disorder. *Journal of Autism and Developmental Disorders, 41*, 1044–1052.

Farley, M. A., McMahon, W. M., Fombonne, E., Jenson, W. R., Miller, J., Gardner, M., et al. (2009). Twenty-year outcome for individuals with autism and average or near-average cognitive abilities. *Autism Research, 2*, 109–118.

Frazier, T. W., Thompson, L., Youngstrom, E. A., Law, P., Hardan, A. Y., Eng, C., & Morris, N. (2014). A twin study of heritable and shared environmental contributions to autism. *Journal of Autism and Developmental Disorders, 44*, 2013–2025.

Green, J., Charman, T., McConachie, H., Aldred, C., Slonims, V., Howlin, P., et al. (2010). Parent-mediated communication-focused treatment in children with autism (PACT): A randomised controlled trial. *The Lancet, 375*, 2152–2160.

Henninger, N. A., & Taylor, J. L. (2013). Outcomes in adults with autism spectrum disorders: A historical perspective. *Autism, 17*, 103–116.

Hess, K. L., Morrier, M. J., Heflin, L. J., & Ivey, M. L. (2008). Autism treatment survey: Services received by children with autism spectrum disorders in public school classrooms. *Journal of Autism and Developmental Disorders, 38*, 961–971.

Howlin, P., Mawhood, L., & Rutter, M. (2000). Autism and developmental receptive language disorder—A follow-up comparison in early adult life. II: Social, behavioural, and psychiatric outcomes. *Journal of Child Psychology and Psychiatry, 41*, 561–578.

Howlin, P., Moss, P., Savage, S., & Rutter, M. (2013). Social outcomes in mid-to later adulthood among individuals diagnosed with autism and average nonverbal IQ as children. *Journal of the American Academy of Child & Adolescent Psychiatry, 52*, 572–581.

Jones, C. R., Happé, F., Golden, H., Marsden, A. J., Tregay, J., Simonoff, E., et al. (2009). Reading and arithmetic in adolescents with autism spectrum disorders: Peaks and dips in attainment. *Neuropsychology, 23*, 718.

Kanner, L. (1943). Autistic disturbances of affective contact. *Nervous Child, 2*, 217–250.

Kasari, C., Lawton, K., Shih, W., Barker, T. V., Landa, R., Lord, C., et al. (2014). Caregiver-mediated intervention for low-resourced preschoolers with autism: An RCT. *Pediatrics, 134*, e72–e79.

Kim, S. H., Bal, V. H., & Lord, C. (2018). Longitudinal follow-up of academic achievement in children with autism from age 2 to 18. *Journal of Child Psychology and Psychiatry, 59*, 258–267.

King, M., & Bearman, P. (2009). Diagnostic change and the increased prevalence of autism. *International Journal of Epidemiology, 38*, 1224–1234.

Kraper, C. K., Kenworthy, L., Popal, H., Martin, A., & Wallace, G. L. (2017). The gap between adaptive behavior and intelligence in autism persists into young adulthood and is linked to psychiatric co-morbidities. *Journal of Autism and Developmental Disorders, 47*, 3007–3017.

Lenoir, P., Bodier, C., Desombre, H., Malvy, J., Abert, B., Ould Taleb, M., & Sauvage, D. (2009). Prevalence of pervasive developmental disorders. A review. *L'Encephale, 35*, 36–42. https://doi.org/10.1016/j.encep.2007.12.011

Lever, A. G., & Geurts, H. M. (2016). Psychiatric co-occurring symptoms and disorders in young, middle-aged, and older adults with autism spectrum disorder. *Journal of Autism and Developmental Disorders, 46*, 1916–1930.

Locke, J., Kasari, C., Rotheram-Fuller, E., Kretzmann, M., & Jacobs, J. (2013). Social network changes over the school year among elementary school-aged children with and without an autism spectrum disorder. *School Mental Health, 5*, 38–47.

Matson, J. L., & Kozlowski, A. M. (2011). The increasing prevalence of autism spectrum disorders. *Research in Autism Spectrum Disorders, 5*, 418–425.

Moseley, D. S., Tonge, B. J., Brereton, A. V., & Einfeld, S. L. (2011). Psychiatric comorbidity in adolescents and young adults with autism. *Journal of Mental Health Research in Intellectual Disabilities, 4*, 229–243.

Newman, L., Wagner, M., Knokey, A. M., Marder, C., Nagle, K., Shaver, D., & Wei, X. (2011). *The post-high school outcomes of young adults with disabilities up to 8 years after high school: A report from the National Longitudinal Transition Study-2 (NLTS2). NCSER 2011-3005.* National Center for Special Education Research.

Orsmond, G. I., Krauss, M. W., & Seltzer, M. M. (2004). Peer relationships and social and recreational activities among adolescents and adults with autism. *Journal of Autism and Developmental Disorders, 34*, 245–256.

Orsmond, G. I., Shattuck, P. T., Cooper, B. P., Sterzing, P. R., & Anderson, K. A. (2013). Social participation among young adults with an autism spectrum disorder. *Journal of Autism and Developmental Disorders, 43*, 2710–2719.

Pandolfi, F., Franza, L., Todi, L., Carusi, V., Centrone, M., Buonomo, A., et al. (2018). The importance of complying with vaccination protocols in developed countries: "Anti-Vax" hysteria and the spread of severe preventable diseases. *Current Medicinal Chemistry, 25*, 6070–6081.
Pennington, M. L., Cullinan, D., & Southern, L. B. (2014). Defining autism: Variability in state education agency definitions of and evaluations for autism spectrum disorders. *Autism Research and Treatment, 2014*, 1–8.
Richa, S., Fahed, M., Khoury, E., & Mishara, B. (2014). Suicide in autism spectrum disorders. *Archives of Suicide Research, 18*, 327–339.
Saito, A., Stickley, A., Haraguchi, H., Takahashi, H., Ishitobi, M., & Kamio, Y. (2017). Association between autistic traits in preschool children and later emotional/behavioral outcomes. *Journal of Autism and Developmental Disorders, 47*, 3333–3346.
Salazar, F., Baird, G., Chandler, S., Tseng, E., O'sullivan, T., Howlin, P., et al. (2015). Co-occurring psychiatric disorders in preschool and elementary school-aged children with autism spectrum disorder. *Journal of Autism and Developmental Disorders, 45*, 2283–2294.
Sanford, C., Newman, L., Wagner, M., Cameto, R., Knokey, A. M., & Shaver, D. (2011). *The post-high school outcomes of young adults with disabilities up to 6 years after high school: Key findings from the National Longitudinal Transition Study-2 (NLTS2). NCSER 2011-3004.* SRI International.
Sealey, L. A., Hughes, B. W., Pestaner, J. P., Steinemann, A., Pace, D. G., & Bagasra, O. (2015). Environmental factors may contribute to autism development and male bias: Effects of fragrances on developing neurons. *Environmental Research, 142*, 731–738.
Tarver, J., Palmer, M., Webb, S., Scott, S., Slonims, V., Simonoff, E., & Charman, T. (2019). Child and parent outcomes following parent interventions for child emotional and behavioral problems in autism spectrum disorders: A systematic review and meta-analysis. *Autism, 23*, 1630–1644.
Taylor, M. J., Rosenqvist, M. A., Larsson, H., Gillberg, C., D'Onofrio, B. M., Lichtenstein, P., & Lundström, S. (2020). Etiology of autism spectrum disorders and autistic traits over time. *JAMA Psychiatry, 77*, 936–943.
Taylor, L. E., Swerdfeger, A. L., & Eslick, G. D. (2014). Vaccines are not associated with autism: An evidence-based meta-analysis of case-control and cohort studies. *Vaccine, 32*, 3623–3629.
Totsika, V., Hastings, R. P., Emerson, E., Berridge, D. M., & Lancaster, G. A. (2011). Behavior problems at 5 years of age and maternal mental health in autism and intellectual disability. *Journal of Abnormal Child Psychology, 39*, 1137–1147.
Treffert, D. A. (1970). Epidemiology of infantile autism. *Archives of General Psychiatry, 22*, 431–438.
Venter, A., Lord, C., & Schopler, E. (1992). A follow-up study of high-functioning autistic children. *Journal of Child Psychology and Psychiatry, 33*, 489–597.
Volkmar, F. R., Scott, L. J., & Hart, L. (2017). Transition issues and challenges for youth with autism spectrum disorders. *Pediatric Annals, 46*, 219–223.
Weiss, J. A., Cappadocia, M. C., Tint, A., & Pepler, D. (2015). Bullying victimization, parenting stress, and anxiety among adolescents and young adults with autism spectrum disorder. *Autism Research, 8*, 727–737.
Whitehouse, A. J., Watt, H. J., Line, E. A., & Bishop, D. V. (2009). Adult psychosocial outcomes of children with specific language impairment, pragmatic language impairment and autism. *International Journal of Language & Communication Disorders, 44*, 511–528.
Whittenburg, H. N., Cimera, R. E., & Thoma, C. A. (2019). Comparing employment outcomes of young adults with autism: Does postsecondary educational experience matter? *Journal of Postsecondary Education and Disability, 32*, 159–172.
Wing, L., & Potter, D. (2002). The epidemiology of autistic spectrum disorders: Is the prevalence rising? *Mental Retardation and Developmental Disabilities Research Reviews, 8*, 151–161.
World Health Organization (WHO). (2019). *The ICD-10 classification of mental and behavioural disorders*. World Health Organization.

Chapter 2
What Are Social Skills?

In order to describe social skills teaching strategies, it is first necessary to define social skills. A variety of definitions have been provided, each focusing on different elements of social skills. Gresham and Elliott (1987) synthesized many of the definitions, describing three primary types of definition: peer acceptance, behavioral or functional, and social validity. Peer acceptance definitions focus on the end product of social interactions—whether an individual is socially accepted or not by their peer group. Individuals who are accepted by their peer group could be said to be socially skilled. Definitions focusing on the end product of social interaction are, however, limited in that they do not describe or define the behaviors associated with social success—thus, they provide little insight into suggested intervention strategies for individuals who present with social skills impairments.

Gresham and Elliott's (1987) second type of definition may ultimately be more useful for intervention development. Behavioral or functional definitions focus on behaviors that result in maximum reinforcement in a particular context while avoiding social punishment. Within a functional or behavioral type of definition, Morgan and Jenson (1988) suggest that social skills may be defined as verbal and nonverbal behaviors that result in a mutually reinforcing social interaction. By definition, reinforcement results in increased future occurrences of a particular behavior. Thus, a mutually reinforcing interaction would be characterized by increased future interactions between the interaction partners or by increased use of a particular social behavior in the future by one of the interaction partners. Although not enumerated, the social skills described in functional or behavioral definitions are specific (i.e., behaviors that result in reinforcement in a particular context), as are the antecedents and consequences of these behaviors—resulting in specific considerations for intervention. Although more useful than a definition based on social acceptance, functional or behavioral definitions are ultimately incomplete in the absence of the final type of definition proposed by Gresham and Elliott (1987)—social validity.

K. C Radley, E. H. Dart, *Social Skills Teaching for Individuals with Autism*, Springer Series on Child and Family Studies,
https://doi.org/10.1007/978-3-030-91665-7_2

Definitions of social skills based on social validity center on the relative social importance of social behaviors in particular context. These types of definitions can be considered to represent a hybrid of social acceptance and functional or behavioral definitions, and emphasize contextual elements. This part of the definition highlights the fact that social skills are ultimately not defined by researchers and practitioners, but are dictated by goals and outcomes that are valued within a particular context. When designing and implementing social skills teaching interventions, researchers and practitioners should focus on these types of definitions—teaching social skills that are related to valued outcomes within a group and that maximize reinforcement within that group.

To illustrate the importance of social validity in defining social skills, one may consider the social skills valued by a group of students. While knowing and using particular terms or slang may not represent a valued outcome to adults or contact positive reinforcement, it may represent skills that are valued by a same-age peer group and result in increased reinforcement and acceptance from said group. Thus, social skill teaching that only emphasizes formal language and interactions may ultimately fall short of being socially valid within a peer group context (i.e., resulting in behaviors that are valued and important within a group). This would, in theory, result in poor skill maintenance and use under real-world situations, decreasing the utility of social skills teaching.

When considering definitions of social skills proposed in the literature, all emphasize the observable nature of social skills. Indeed, social skills should be conceptualized as discrete social behaviors. Social skills are related to, but differentiated from, social competence through their discrete and observable nature. Social competence can be defined as judgments regarding an individual's social skill or performance (Hops, 1983) or the ability of an individual to successfully adapt their social skills to a given context (e.g., Semrud-Clikeman, 2007). Social skills, however, should be conceptualized as the discrete behaviors through which social competence is demonstrated. Given that social skills represent discrete behaviors, it is therefore possible to develop ecologically validated task analyses of social skills.

Socially and Culturally Dependent

Although not emphasized in any of the previously described definitions, it is critical to note that social skills are behaviors that are learned and acquired through interaction with one's environment. Gresham and Elliott (1984) and Cook et al. (2008) specifically identify that social skills are learned behaviors that facilitate social interaction. Ladd (2005) expands upon the notion of learned behaviors, indicating that these behaviors are culturally associated. This distinction is meaningful, in that it emphasizes the lack of universality of social skills and the need to consider cultural and contextual variables when planning and implementing social skills teaching interventions. The lack of universality of social skills is even apparent within cultural groups, whereas members of a particular cultural background may share some characteristics with respect to social skills, other elements (e.g., age, gender, SES) also influence social behaviors that are valued and reinforced within a group.

Given the multiple influences on social behavior, it is therefore necessary that practitioners adopt flexibility in defining and teaching social skills. Effective social skills teaching is contingent upon comprehensive assessment of an individual's environment. Further, social skills teaching should rely on stakeholder input to identify and define target skills—increasing social validity of skills taught within an intervention and identifying skills that will contact naturally reinforcing contingencies across environments in which the individual interacts with others. The goal of social skills teaching should not be that all individuals demonstrate skills that conform to a standard set by one group of individuals, but that individuals utilize skills that will help them be maximally successful across environments (Cartledge & Loe, 2001).

What Social Skills Are Not

The previous paragraphs have defined essential elements of social skills: functional (i.e., result in reinforcement and avoid punishment), socially valid, discrete, and learned and culturally mediated behaviors. Although commonly identified as social skills, constructs such as empathy and respect fail to meet the aforementioned elements of social skills. Although development of empathy and respect are notable objectives, they do not represent discrete and observable behaviors. Instead, such constructs are likely to be more similar to the construct of social competence, in which discrete social behaviors represent individual components within the broader construct of empathy and respect. For example, demonstration of empathy may, at times, consist of more discrete behaviors such as recognizing emotions of others, asking how others are feeling, or expressing support of others.

By the same token, broad or poorly defined classes of behavior also fail to meet the definition of social skills. For example, "communication skills" should not be considered a social skill as it, too, may comprise multiple discrete social behaviors (e.g., requesting information or help, initiating or terminating an interaction). Indeed, considering broad classes of social behaviors is important and has potential social significance. For example, Little et al. (2019) suggest seven broad classes of social skills that are related to positive outcomes: communication, cooperation, assertion, responsibility, empathy, engagement, and self-control. However, improvement in these areas should be considered to be goals, as they relate to broad and abstract areas; instead, social skills teaching must focus on specific and measurable objectives—defined as the discrete social behaviors which may comprise the broader goals.

Outcomes of Social Behavior

Social skills teaching represents one of the most common intervention strategies for intervention with ASD in both research (e.g., Palmen et al., 2012) and applied settings (e.g., Hess et al., 2008). The frequency with which social skills teaching is utilized is likely due to the well documented proximal and distal outcomes of effective use of social skills.

Proximal Outcomes

Effective use of social skills is associated with a number of positive and immediate outcomes for individuals. For example, effective social skill use is associated with decreased isolation and greater social connectedness among peer groups (e.g., Kasari et al., 2016). They are also associated with demonstration of effective communication and play skills (e.g., Barnett, 2018). Poor social skills may also be associated with poorer quality teacher–student relationships for individuals with ASD (Blacher et al., 2014). Individuals with poor social skills report less frequent contact with peers and decreased participation in social interactions outside of school (e.g., Wagner et al., 2003) and other community events (Myers et al., 2015).

Distal Outcomes

A range of poor long-term outcomes are associated with poor social skill use. For example, poor social skills are related to increased anxiety and depression in individuals with ASD (White et al., 2007). Related to mental health, poor social functioning is associated with increased suicidality (e.g., Van Meter et al., 2019). Poor social skill use is also related to increased risk of victimization and exploitation (Humphrey & Symes, 2010; Sullivan & Caterino, 2008). Social competence represents a critical domain for obtaining and maintaining employment (Agran et al., 2016), with social skill use being predictive of postsecondary employment (Chiang et al., 2013). Additional researchers have documented the positive effect of social skills on postsecondary employment, as well as participation in postsecondary education and increased functional independence (Nasamran et al., 2017).

Social Skills Deficits

As mentioned in the previous chapter, deficits in social communication are one of the defining features of ASD. A comparison of the social skills profiles of individuals with ASD to those without revealed substantial differences in their verbal and nonverbal social behavior (Wilkins & Matson, 2009) supporting the idea that deficits in social behavior are central to ASD. A social skills deficit is an individual's lack of knowledge about how a specific social behavior should be exhibited and under which circumstances or a lack of performance of a known skill under the expected circumstances. Social skills deficits can be broad, covering many discrete skills (e.g., appropriate facial expressions, tone of voice, expressing wants and needs, requesting help, initiating, maintaining, and terminating conversations), or narrow, impacting just one specific skill (e.g., asking someone out on a date). In either case, the nature of the deficit must be identified.

Prior to beginning a social skills teaching program, it is critical to consider whether an identified social deficit is due to a lack of skill acquisition or low motivation to perform an already learned skill. Acquisition deficits reflect a lack of understanding in how the skill or behavior should be performed. For example, if an individual does not know how to terminate a conversation appropriately, they are likely to do so in a manner that is awkward, abrupt, or inappropriate (e.g., exhibit aggression). On the other hand, performance deficits reflect a lack of motivation to exhibit a skill due to competing contingencies of reinforcement operating on other behaviors. For example, an individual may know how to terminate a conversation appropriately but instead may choose to engage in aggressive behavior because it has historically resulted in more immediate termination of any ongoing conversation. Although the particular deficit in these examples may appear topographically identical (i.e., aggressive behavior to terminate a conversation), the distinction between acquisition deficits and performance deficits holds important practical considerations. Thus, it is critical to engage in assessment to determine whether a particular social skills deficit is one of acquisition or performance.

There are several methods that can be used to determine whether a social skill deficit is acquisition based or performance based. Gresham and colleagues (2010) examined the base rates of both among a very large sample of children ages 3 through 18 and found that acquisition deficits were quite rare (i.e., <1% of sample). Performance deficits were more common, with at least 50% of the sample exhibiting at least one performance-based deficit. Although no comparable study of children with ASD exists, the importance of identifying the nature of social skills deficits remains (Bellini et al., 2007). Conducting observations of an individual's naturalistic social behavior or interviewing them or individuals in their environment may be a valuable source of information. Looking for or asking about whether specific social skills have been exhibited would shed light on whether the individual possesses the skill and is motivated to exhibit it.

A more direct approach might involve conducting assessments of an individual's social behavior. Duhon et al. (2004) first describe an assessment technique that could be used to determine the nature of an academic skill deficit (Duhon et al., 2004). The technique involved assessing a student's academic skill performance (e.g., oral reading fluency) two times, once to determine a present level of performance, and again to determine if the individual could be motivated to surpass their present level. A reinforcement contingency was used to increase motivation to perform (e.g., "You read 40 words the first time, if you can beat your score this time you'll earn a prize!"). Logically, if an individual is able to substantially increase their performance in the brief time between the two assessments, the difference can be attributed to a performance deficit; however, if the individual's performance does not improve even under the reinforcement contingency, the deficit can be attributed to an acquisition deficit. This assessment method could also be applied to social skills. An individual could be prompted to exhibit a specific skill (e.g., initiating a conversation) and, if a deficit is present, be offered the opportunity to try again for an incentive if they are able to exhibit the skill accurately or more appropriately. Just as with students' academic skills, if an individual can exhibit more appropriate social behavior in a short time span when incentivized, the deficit is likely performance based. Otherwise, it is likely safe to assume that the individual does not know how to perform the skill appropriately (i.e., acquisition deficit).

Once the nature of the social skills deficit has been identified, it is possible to begin developing an appropriate treatment plan that will be used to teach the skill (i.e., acquisition deficit), promote skill use (i.e., performance deficit), or both.

Teaching and Measuring

Before any social skills assessment, teaching, or other intervention work can begin, it is important to identify and define the skill or skills of interest. As discussed earlier in this chapter, social skills should be conceptualized as discrete behaviors (e.g., greeting, initiating a conversation, requesting assistance) and not broad or subjective constructs (e.g., social emotional competence, emotional intelligence, empathy). When conceptualized in this way, the most sensitive assessment method to monitor acquisition and performance of social skills will be direct observation of a learner's performance of the skill. Although there are many standardized and criterion-referenced rating scales available (e.g., Stone et al., 2003; Bellini & Hopf, 2007; Gresham et al., 2011) to assess and individual's social skills, we recommend reserving these assessments for long-term summative evaluation of learner progress. Direct observation of learner performance can be conducted daily and, as will be described later, sensitive to changes in skill acquisition and performance on a trial-by-trial basis. These data can then be used to make determinations about whether a skill deficit exists and monitors individuals' response to interventions.

Before direct observation can be conducted, it is necessary to develop an operational definition for each skill to be assessed. Operational definitions are clear, concise, and complete descriptions of a behavior that can be used to determine whether a behavior did or did not occur (Furlow, 2018). Operational definitions should be unambiguous such that two individuals observing the same behavior could both agree that the behavior was or was not exhibited. Because social skills involve interacting with others, it will likely be necessary to include any relevant antecedent conditions that set the occasion for appropriate skill use. Further, because social behaviors are sometimes complex and involve multiple steps, it is common to develop task analyses to aid in their assessment.

Like operational definitions, task analyses provide clear and concise descriptions of behavior; however, unlike operational definitions, they specify a sequence in which a chain of behaviors must be completed. Task analyses are used frequently in social skills intervention work because they allow an observer to determine whether each step of a complex social behavior was exhibited appropriately and in the correct order. Creating a task analysis involves identifying the essential elements of the specific skill to be addressed and arranging them in the appropriate sequence. Commercially published social skills curricula (e.g., Skillstreaming; Goldstein & McGinnis, 1997) provide task analyses for the social skills included within the program; however, it may be desirable to create your own task analyses in the event that (1) you do not have access to any curricula, (2) you want to assess a skill that is not covered in existing curricula, or (3) you want to ensure that your task analysis is relevant to your learners. When developing a task analysis for social skill assessment and intervention, consider recruiting input from relevant stakeholders such as caregivers, clients, and community members. As mentioned previously, social behavior is contextual and dependent on environmental factors and cultural norms. Collaboratively developing task analyses and operational definitions may enhance the social validity of the work and promote generalization and maintenance of skill use once teaching is complete.

Combining both operational definitions and tasks analyses allows for a complete and comprehensive description of the discrete behavior being assessed. Once your task analysis and operational definitions are developed, you can use them to assess social skill acquisition and performance across settings.

Acquisition Assessing the acquisition of a social skill by a learner involves comparing their performance of the skill to the task analysis and recording which steps were exhibited accurately and which were not. That is, each attempt by the learner to exhibit the skill is considered a trial and performance in that trial is evaluated on a step-by-step basis. Acquisition of the skill would be evidenced by an individual's consistent and accurate demonstration of the skill. Figure 2.1 depicts how acquisition data might be presented on a trial-by-trial basis. That is, each opportunity to perform the skill is plotted as a separate data point with the percentage of task analysis steps exhibited accurately reflected on the *y*-axis. These data depict a short pre-treatment phase with low accuracy, followed by rapid acquisition of the skill and ending with three consecutive trials of 100% accuracy. Alternatively, if learners are given multiple opportunities to exhibit the skill within a teaching session, it may be desirable to reflect acquisition as the percentage of trials in which 100% accuracy was achieved. Figure 2.2 depicts an example of session-by-session data wherein a learner was given ten opportunities to exhibit a social skill per session. A short pre-treatment phase depicts two sessions with a single trial at mastery and three sessions with no trials at mastery. Once treatment begins, rapid acquisition is observed and the phase ends with three consecutive sessions with 100% of trials at mastery.

Performance Once a social skill has been acquired by a learner, assessment of their performance of the skill in novel environments is recommended to determine if their learning generalizes across settings, people, or antecedent stimuli. To do this, it is

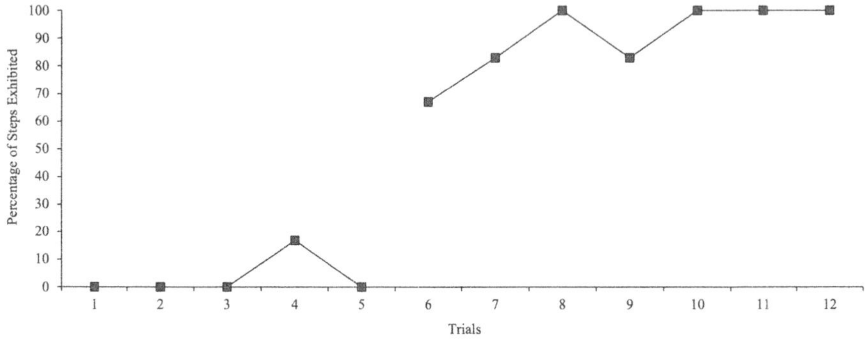

Fig. 2.1 Graphed data depicting social skill acquisition by trial using a task analysis

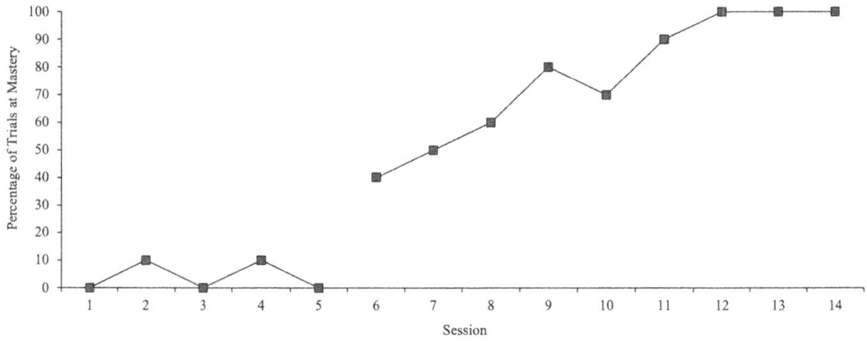

Fig. 2.2 Graphed data depicting social skill acquisition by session using a task analysis

critical to examine frequency of skill performance in addition to accuracy. Figure 2.3 depicts a graph of a learner's combined accuracy and performance data. The line portion of the graph, plotted on the left-hand *y*-axis, depicts the frequency with which the learner attempted to initiate social interactions during each session. The bars behind the line, plotted on the right-hand *y*-axis, depict the percentage of initiations that were exhibited at mastery for each session. As can be seen, the first five sessions depict a decreasing trend in frequency but an increasing trend in accuracy. The onset of a performance-deficit intervention resulted in an increase in the frequency of social interactions as well as more consistency in accuracy. Using both pieces of data allows for a complete assessment of the frequency with which a learner exhibits a skill as well as the accuracy with which they do so.

Conclusion

In closing, we want to emphasize that assessment and treatment of social communication deficits in individuals with ASD begin with a clear conceptualization of social behavior as many discrete, and sometimes complex, skills. Developing

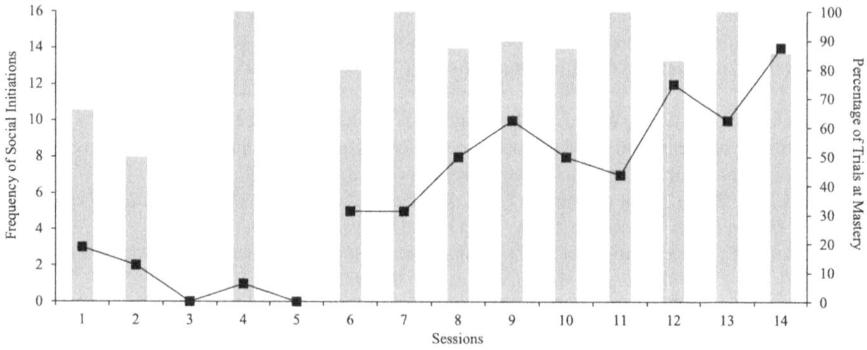

Fig. 2.3 Graphed data depicting social skill performance

concrete operational definitions and complete task analyses for each skill is a critical first step in the assessment and intervention process. Monitoring skill acquisition and performance is most sensitive when using direct observation of skill use; however, rating scales may be useful for summarizing long-term change from various stakeholders. The remainder of this book will describe evidence-based intervention strategies that can be used to remediate social skill acquisition and performance deficits in individuals with ASD. Each chapter will cover a specific strategy, ordered by the frequency with which they appear in the scholarly literature (Radley et al., 2020).

References

Agran, M., Hughes, C., Thoma, C. A., & Scott, L. A. (2016). Employment social skills: What skills are really valued? *Career Development and Transition for Exceptional Individuals, 39*, 111–120.

Barnett, J. H. (2018). Three evidence-based strategies that support social skills and play among young children with autism spectrum disorders. *Early Childhood Education Journal, 46*(6), 665–672.

Bellini, S., & Hopf, A. (2007). The development of the Autism Social Skills Profile: A preliminary analysis of psychometric properties. *Focus on Autism and Other Developmental Disabilities, 22*, 80–87.

Bellini, S., Peters, J. K., Benner, L., & Hopf, A. (2007). A meta-analysis of school-based social skills interventions for children with autism spectrum disorders. *Remedial and Special Education, 28*, 153–162.

Blacher, J., Howell, E., Lauderdale-Littin, S., Reed, F. D. D., & Laugeson, E. A. (2014). Autism spectrum disorder and the student teacher relationship: A comparison study with peers with intellectual disability and typical development. *Research in Autism Spectrum Disorders, 8*, 324–333.

Cartledge, G., & Loe, S. A. (2001). Cultural diversity and social skill instruction. *Exceptionality, 9*, 33–46.

Chiang, H. M., Cheung, Y. K., Li, H., & Tsai, L. Y. (2013). Factors associated with participation in employment for high school leavers with autism. *Journal of Autism and Developmental Disorders, 43*, 1832–1842.

Cook, C. R., Gresham, F. M., Kern, L., Barreras, R. B., Thornton, S., & Crews, S. D. (2008). Social skills training for secondary students with emotional and/or behavioral disorders: A review and analysis of the meta-analytic literature. *Journal of Emotional and Behavioral Disorders, 16*, 131–144.
Duhon, G. J., Noell, G. H., Witt, J. C., Freeland, J. T., Dufrene, B. A., & Gilbertson, D. N. (2004). Identifying academic skill and performance deficits: The experimental analysis of brief assessments of academic skills. *School Psychology Review, 33*, 429–443.
Furlow, C. M. (2018). What is behavior? In K. C. Radley & E. H. Dart (Eds.), *Handbook of behavioral interventions in schools* (pp. 1–14). Oxford University Press.
Goldstein, A. P., & McGinnis, E. (1997). *Skill streaming the Adolescents: New strategies and perspectives for teaching prosocial skills* (Rev. ed.). Research Press.
Gresham, F. M., & Elliott, S. N. (1984). Assessment and classification of children's social skills: A review of methods and issues. *School Psychology Review, 13*, 292–301.
Gresham, F. M., & Elliott, S. N. (1987). The relationship between adaptive behavior and social skills: Issues in definition and assessment. *The Journal of Special Education, 21*, 167–181.
Gresham, F. M., Elliott, S. N., & Kettler, R. J. (2010). Base rates of social skills acquisition/performance deficits, strengths, and problem behaviors: An analysis of the Social Skills Improvement System—Rating Scales. *Psychological Assessment, 22*, 809.
Gresham, F. M., Elliott, S. N., Vance, M. J., & Cook, C. R. (2011). Comparability of the social skills rating system to the social skills improvement system: Content and psychometric comparisons across elementary and secondary age levels. *School Psychology Quarterly, 26*, 27–44.
Hess, K. L., Morrier, M. J., Heflin, L. J., & Ivey, M. L. (2008). Autism treatment survey: Services received by children with autism spectrum disorders in public school classrooms. *Journal of Autism and Developmental Disorders, 38*, 961–971.
Hops, H. (1983). Children's social competence and skill: Current research practices and future directions. *Behavior Therapy, 14*, 3–18.
Humphrey, N., & Symes, W. (2010). Responses to bullying and use of social support among pupils with autism spectrum disorders (ASDs) in mainstream schools: A qualitative study. *Journal of Research in Special Educational Needs, 10*, 82–90.
Kasari, C., Dean, M., Kretzmann, M., Shih, W., Orlich, F., Whitney, R., Landa, R., Lord, C., & King, B. (2016). Children with autism spectrum disorder and social skills groups at school: A randomized trial comparing intervention approach and peer composition. *The Journal of Child Psychology and Psychiatry, 57*, 171–179.
Ladd, G. W. (2005). *Children's peer relations and social competence: A century of progress*. Yale University Press.
Little, S. G., Akin-Little, A., Gopaul, M., & Nicholson, T. (2019). Social skills. In *Handbook of intellectual disabilities* (pp. 685–697).
Morgan, D. P., & Jenson, W. R. (1988). *Teaching behaviorally disordered students: Preferred practices*. Merrill Publishing Co.
Myers, E., Davis, B. E., Stobbe, G., & Bjornson, K. (2015). Community and social participation among individuals with autism spectrum disorder transitioning to adulthood. *Journal of Autism and Developmental Disorders, 45*, 2373–2381.
Nasamran, A., Witmer, S. E., & Los, J. E. (2017). Exploring predictors of postsecondary outcomes for students with autism spectrum disorder. *Education and Training in Autism and Developmental Disabilities, 52*, 343–356.
Palmen, A., Didden, R., & Lang, R. (2012). A systematic review of behavioral intervention research on adaptive skill building in high-functioning young adults with autism spectrum disorder. *Research in Autism Spectrum Disorders, 6*, 602–617.
Radley, K. C., Dart, E. H., Brennan, K. J., Helbig, K. A., Lehman, E. L., Silberman, M., & Mendanhall, K. (2020). Social skills teaching for individuals with autism spectrum disorder: A systematic review. *Advances in Neurodevelopmental Disorders, 4*, 215–226.
Semrud-Clikeman, M. (2007). Social competence in children. In *Social competence in children* (pp. 1–9). Springer.

Stone, W., Ruble, L., Coonrod, E., Hepburn, S., Pennington, M., Burnette, C., & Brigham, N. B. (2003). *TRIAD social skills assessment manual*. Treatment and Research Institute for Autism Spectrum Disorders.

Sullivan, A., & Caterino, L. C. (2008). Addressing the sexuality and sex education of individuals with autism spectrum disorders. *Education and Treatment of Children, 31*(3), 381–394.

Van Meter, A. R., Paksarian, D., & Merikangas, K. R. (2019). Social functioning and suicide risk in a community sample of adolescents. *Journal of Clinical Child & Adolescent Psychology, 48*, 273–287.

Wagner, M., Cadwallader, T., Marder, C., Cameto, R., Cardoso, D., Garza, N., Levine, P., & Newman, L. (2003). Life outside the classroom for youth with disabilities. In *A report from the National Longitudinal Transition Study-2 (NLTS2)*. SRI International.

White, S. W., Keonig, K., & Scahill, L. (2007). Social skills development in children with autism spectrum disorders: A review of the intervention research. *Journal of Autism and Developmental Disorders, 37*, 1858–1868.

Wilkins, J., & Matson, J. L. (2009). A comparison of social skills profiles in intellectually disabled adults with and without ASD. *Behavior Modification, 33*, 143–155.

Chapter 3
Video Modeling

Video modeling (VM) primarily involves having a learner watch a recorded video of an individual exhibiting a specific social skill appropriately and usually within the relevant social context. Because the primary component of VM is a depiction of appropriate skill use, it is generally considered an intervention strategy used to address acquisition deficits rather than performance deficits; however, we will describe later how other components are sometimes included in video models to extend their reach to address both types of social skills deficits. At a theoretical level, VM capitalizes on social learning theory to promote treatment effects.

Social learning theory (Bandura & McClelland, 1977), itself based in behavioral learning theory (Skinner, 1963), posits that individuals can learn to engage in behaviors not only through their own interaction with their environment but by observing others interacting with their environment as well. Through operant conditioning, human behavior is selected and shaped by its consequences, meaning we are more likely to re-exhibit behaviors that contact pleasant consequences and less likely to re-exhibit behaviors that contact unpleasant consequences. Bandura's social learning theory extended this idea by proposing that observing the operant conditioning process at work on others' behavior has similar effects. That is, we are more or less likely to engage in the behaviors we observe exhibited by others depending on whether we perceive the consequences of their behavior to be pleasant or unpleasant, respectively.

This proposal garnered experimental evidence when Bandura (1965) demonstrated that children who observed a video model being punished (i.e., social disapproval) for exhibiting aggressive behavior toward an inflatable doll were themselves less likely to exhibit aggressive behavior toward the doll. Further, an increase in aggressive behavior toward the doll was exhibited by all experimental groups when children were incentivized to mimic the model's behavior, regardless of whether the model was punished, reinforced, or experienced no consequences. The results of this seminal study support the idea that humans are sensitive to the consequences of

K. C Radley, E. H. Dart, *Social Skills Teaching for Individuals with Autism*, Springer Series on Child and Family Studies,
https://doi.org/10.1007/978-3-030-91665-7_3

others' behavior and are able to exhibit modeled behavior when their environment is arranged to reinforce such behavior. These findings set the stage for decades of research on VM as a treatment strategy to promote social skills acquisition and performance in individuals with ASD.

One of the earliest examples of video modeling to teach social skills with this population was conducted by Charlop and Milstein (1989). Previously, others had used video modeling to teach adaptive behaviors (i.e., purchasing items from a store; Haring et al., 1987) but this study represents the first demonstration of its use to target learner acquisition of social behavior. Charlop and Milstein (1989) created video models of brief conversations (i.e., 45 s) between two adults about toys and activities relevant to the learners' interests. Learners were then engaged in conversations identical to the ones they observed in the models and their responses were evaluated for correctness and novelty. All three child participants with ASD exhibited increases in appropriate conversation skills following the video modeling procedure. Additionally, generalization across settings, toys and activities, and conversants was observed. This study set the stage for over three decades of subsequent VM literature and the practice is now considered an evidence-based strategy.

Empirical Basis of VM

In 2009, the May Institute's National Autism Center's National Standards Project identified modeling (including VM) as an evidence-based strategy to promote beneficial effects within the domain's communication and interpersonal behaviors for individuals with ASD ages 3–18 (CITE). This classification was reaffirmed in Phase 2 of the National Standards Project (CITE). Although the evidence-based designation depends somewhat on the standards that have been adopted to make such determinations, the National Standards Project criteria for effective treatments are rigorous and provide strong support for VM. A systematic review conducted by Qi et al. (2018) also concluded that VM was an evidence-based practice according to the What Works Clearinghouse criteria. Additionally, two quantitative syntheses of the peer-reviewed literature also provide additional support for video modeling specifically.

Bellini and Akullian (2007) synthesized the results of 23 studies investigating video modeling and video-self modeling (VSM), in which the model in the video is the learner, and described the strategies as moderately effective (Percentage of Nonoverlapping Data [PND] = 80%, range = 29–100). They also examined the two as separate strategies and found small differences in treatment effect between VM (PND = 88%) and VSM (PND = 71%); however, they did note that generalization of treatment effects was more pronounced for VM over VSM, suggesting that the incorporation of others into video models may confer additional benefits. Finally, Bellini and Akullian (2007) examined the effectiveness of both strategies when used specifically to promote social communication and found it moderately effective

(PND = 77%) compared to its use to promote adaptive behavior (PND = 89%) and other behaviors (PND = 76%).

More recently, Wang et al. (2011) employed more complex statistical analyses to synthesize and compare the literature supporting VM and peer-mediated strategies to address social skills of youth with ASD. After a systematic literature review, five VM studies were included in the meta-analysis along with nine peer-mediated strategies. Across all 14 studies, the average standardized treatment effect was 1.27, suggesting a strong impact on social behavior. Wang and colleagues reported that while treatment type (i.e., VM vs. peer-mediated) did not significantly predict effect size, the age of participants did. Specifically, they found that the effectiveness of VM interventions were sensitive to participant age, with those aimed at younger children more effective than those aimed at older children and adolescents. Taken together, the endorsement from the National Autism Center and these two meta-analyses provide strong general support for VM as an intervention strategy to promote social skill acquisition in individuals with ASD.

Radley et al.' (2020) systematic review of interventions to promote social behavior in individuals with ASD identified VM and VSM as the most well-researched strategy in this area. Consistent with its primary function as a skill acquisition intervention, they noted that over half of all VM studies focused on acquisition as the primary target of the intervention; however, the remaining studies examined social engagement as an outcome, suggesting it also serves to promote performance of skills in context. Additionally, they noted that the average participant age in VM studies is 6.9, suggesting it is primarily used with younger children, consistent with the recommendations made in Wang et al.' (2011) meta-analytic synthesis. VM may not be appropriate for learners who do not have the sensory (e.g., visual impairments) or cognitive capacity to attend to the video content.

Implementation Examples from the Literature

Next, to provide examples of how video modeling is typically practiced, we will review the procedures of two VM studies. The first, by Miltenberger and Charlop (2015), compared two modes of VM delivery (i.e., traditional television vs. tablet computer) to determine whether either promoted more rapid acquisition of social behaviors across five participants. The second, by Lee et al. (2017) was conducted with a single participant and used VSM to promote three functional play skills.

Miltenberger and Charlop (2015) created videos with adult models exhibiting social skills that were idiosyncratically selected across five participants (i.e., conversational speech, pretend play, interactive play, asking questions, requesting). Each video consisted of the adult model looking into the camera and "demonstrated speech and nonverbal behavior at an exaggeratedly slow pace" (Miltenberger & Charlop, 2015, p. 344). To begin each treatment session, participants would watch the video model either on the television or tablet computer, and then enter a testing session during which they would be asked to demonstrate the behavior they observed in the video. These sessions were held in a variety of locations (e.g., cafe, outdoors, clinic room) to assess generalization. Miltenberger and Charlop (2015) found that skill acquisition was generally more rapid when a television was used to present the video model; however, generalization of skills was more pronounced for those skills taught using the VM presented with the tablet computer. Additionally, the latency between VM presentation and test session was briefer in the tablet computer condition, due to its portability and ease of use.

Lee et al. (2017) identified six functional play behaviors each across three sets of toys and used VSM to promote acquisition and performance of the behaviors with a 5-year-old child with ASD. To create the VSM, the researchers filmed the participant playing with each toy set across three different days and prompted him to engage in each of the functional play behaviors. The video footage was then edited to create three separate video models, one per play set. Each video model lasted approximately 45 s and began with an introduction (e.g., "This is Ryan's movie, starring Ryan. Let's watch Ryan play with the farm toys." p. 2299). Statements of praise by the researchers would follow each play behavior exhibited by the participant in the video and each video was doubled so that it played through all six behaviors two times. Each video was approximately 2 min long. At the start of each treatment session, the participant would be asked to watch a video, the VSM would be played, and he would then be prompted to engage with the play set featured in the video. The results of the study supported rapid acquisition of the play behaviors featured in the VSM with maintenance of the behaviors evident over a 2-week follow-up period.

These two studies represent a small fraction of the VM and VSM literature available but hopefully provide a more concrete picture of how this strategy can be used to promote social behavior in children with ASD. Next, we will describe a comprehensive guide to create, edit, and employ VMs in practical settings.

Guide to Practice

When considering implementing a video modeling intervention to teach social skills, three factors should be considered: learners, stakeholders, and resources (Collier-Meek et al., 2012). These factors, described in more detail below, are critical to the determination of whether a video modeling intervention may be appropriate for a particular learner.

Learner Factors

First, an interventionist must consider whether a video modeling intervention would meet the needs of the learner. In order to do so, it is necessary that the interventionist have comprehensive and multi-informant data regarding the social functioning of the learner. Ideally, these data should provide the interventionist with information regarding the type of social skill deficit that a learner may have and document any interfering behaviors. These data are useful in determining whether additional supports are needed (e.g., reinforcement strategies for skill use) or the content that should be depicted in the video model (e.g., labeling of discrete skill steps). Data should also describe settings in which the target skill should be utilized, as video models should demonstrate skill use in similar settings as a means of promoting generalization of the skill from the teaching context.

As video modeling entails a learner viewing a video of skill use, the ability to attend to a video should be considered a prerequisite skill (e.g., Dowrick, 1999). The potential for a learner to demonstrate the target skill should also be a primary factor in electing video modeling as an intervention modality. For example, use of a vocal greeting (e.g., "How's it going?") would require a learner to be able to communicate vocally. A video model demonstrating vocal greetings would therefore be inappropriate and ultimately ineffective for a learner with a limited vocal repertoire. It is not critical for a student to be able to demonstrate a target skill independently for video modeling to be used; however, interventionists should ensure that a learner can demonstrate all steps to a skill with coaching or prompting. Finally, interventionists should consult the literature to determine the extent to which similar social skills have been addressed using video modeling (Collier-Meek et al., 2012). Although the research broadly supports the efficacy of video modeling (e.g., McCoy & Hermansen, 2007), the extant literature should provide a guide for specific procedures and video modeling variations that may be most effective for a particular learner (Collier-Meek et al., 2012).

Stakeholder Factors

Stakeholder buy-in is a critical element to intervention fidelity and effectiveness. As such, when considering implementation of a video modeling intervention, interventionists should consider the perception that stakeholders may have of video modeling. If practitioners view the intervention as unneeded, overly time consuming or burdensome, or likely to be ineffective, video modeling may not be utilized as intended or with the recommended dosage—resulting in an intervention that is less effective and likely to reinforce unfavorable attitudes toward the intervention. As a means of improving buy-in, interventionists should clearly describe intervention procedures and perceived challenges with stakeholders, adapting the intervention to fit the needs of the student and the capacity of the stakeholder to implement the intervention while maintaining the integrity of the intervention procedures (e.g., Sanetti et al., 2015). Even in the absence of stakeholder resistance, interventionists should ensure that stakeholders have the requisite capacities (e.g., training, resources) to be able to implement the intervention as intended—providing the requisite support to ensure that the intervention may be implemented with fidelity.

Resource Factors

Common technology (e.g., smart phones equipped with cameras and video editing apps) has reduced resource burdens previously associated with video modeling (e.g., need for camera, video editing software). However, other resources must still be considered—particularly with respect to time to plan, record, and edit the video model. Interventionists must also be aware of personnel needs associated with the video model. Whereas some video modeling strategies include the learner themselves (i.e., video self-modeling), others may provide demonstrations of skill use by individuals other than the learner or depict interactions between the learner and communication partners. In these cases, it is critical that interventionists plan for additional personnel within a video model and ensure that appropriate consent and assent is obtained prior to inclusion of such individuals.

Implementing Video Modeling

Collier-Meek et al. (2012) describe a ten-step procedure for producing video models, consisting of the following: planning and preparation for the intervention, obtaining parental permission, working with a collaborative team, developing operational definitions, collecting baseline data and identifying target levels of behavior, considering logistical issues, videotaping, editing, presenting the video model to the learner, and evaluating outcomes. These steps, described in more detail below, provide a comprehensive guide to video modeling. However, it should be noted that several variations of video modeling exist and have been found to be beneficial (e.g., video self-modeling, feedforward); thus, some procedural variations are likely to exist within the steps described below.

Plan

As previously described, several considerations should first be made prior to designing and implementing a video modeling intervention. In particular, it is critical that video modeling be identified as appropriate for the learner and target skill, with interventionists consulting the empirical literature to identify exemplars of video modeling that are similar to their planned use of the strategy.

Permission

Following determination that video modeling is an appropriate strategy, the interventionist should obtain permission to implement the intervention with the learner. Collier-Meek et al. (2012) suggest that consent for video modeling should clearly describe the process of producing the video model, including filming, editing, storage and security, and use of the intervention. In addition to obtaining consent for the learner, the interventionist must also obtain consent for all other individuals that may appear in the video model. For example, if a video model will depict a conflict resolution skill, it may be important to include a similarly aged peer—necessitating obtaining consent for that individual to appear in the video model. Finally, interventionists should consider whether assent of the learner or others that may appear in the video is required.

Collaboration

As described in previous chapters, social skills should be conceptualized contextually and based on their social validity. As such, it is critical that interventionists collaborate with stakeholders to ensure that the target social skill is socially valid and contextually representative of skill use in environments in which the learner interacts with others. Stakeholders may include, but are not limited to, caregivers, teachers, interventionists (e.g., psychologists, counselors), administrators, and the students themselves. In addition to ensuring the social validity of the skills to be addressed, this group should work to identify processes, goals, and context of the intervention (Sheridan et al., 2010), ensuring clarity of roles and function of each individual as part of the intervention—a process that is likely to result in greater integrity and satisfaction with intervention procedures.

Operational Definitions

During collaboration with stakeholders, operational definitions of target social skills should be developed. Operational definitions must describe discrete skill use and pass the Stranger Test, in which an individual unfamiliar with the learner would be able to discriminate between occurrences and non-occurrences of the target behavior using only the written description of the skill.

Data Collection

Measurement of present levels of social skills functioning is critical to any social skills teaching intervention. Following development of operational definitions, data collection should commence in a manner that produces valid estimates of the skills defined. A variety of dimensions should be considered as relevant dimensions of social skills, including duration, latency, frequency, and intensity of behaviors (e.g., Gresham, 2001). Applying these dimensions to social skills teaching, an interventionist may assess the duration of social engagement via continuous measurement (e.g., number of seconds of interaction) or discontinuous methods (e.g., momentary time sampling; Cooper et al., 2020). Interventionists in applied settings should aim to collect data in a similar manner to research with respect to frequency of data collection prior to—allowing stakeholders to accurately conceptualize present levels of functioning and set goals for intervention. The same level of intensity of data collection should be continued throughout the intervention, providing stakeholders with sufficient data to evaluate learner response to intervention.

Logistics

Prior to creating and implementing video models, Collier-Meek et al. (2012) suggest developing a schedule for filming, editing, presenting video models, and collecting data during the intervention period. The process of creating a schedule should be done with the intent of removing ambiguity regarding timelines and roles of stakeholders within the intervention process. During logistical planning, stakeholders should review technological requirements and test equipment to ensure that the intervention can be completed as intended. Collier-Meek et al. (2012) also suggest reviewing procedures for maintaining privacy and confidentiality of learners, ensuring that intervention materials are appropriately protected and to protect against loss of intervention materials or data.

Filming

Researchers have primarily utilized one of three types of video modeling: video modeling, in which a known or unknown individual demonstrates accurate skill use via video; video self-modeling, in which the learner demonstrates accurate skill use via video; and feedforward, in which the learner is prompted to demonstrate a skill accurately and video editing is utilized to depict accurate and prompt-free skill use. Other researchers have varied the perspective of the video, using first- or third-person video. Although each of these types of video modeling would entail different filming procedures, some general considerations should be made regardless of the type of video modeling utilized.

First, video models should depict best examples of target skill use. Although inaccurate video models may be used to provide a learner with opportunities to identify errors in skill use, all video models should demonstrate complete and accurate skill use. Second, video models should be filmed in naturalistic locations, a technique likely to enhance the generalization of social skills from training settings to generalized settings (e.g., Stokes & Baer, 1977). Third, videos should demonstrate multiple exemplars of skills. If skills are to be used across multiple persons and settings, video models should aim to provide models of skill use under those conditions.

Editing

Once filmed, the video model should be edited to ensure that best demonstrations of the target skill are represented in the final product. The final video modeling materials should be 2–5 min in duration (Hitchcock et al., 2003)—providing sufficient time to depict multiple models of accurate skill use without losing interest or attention of the learner (Collier-Meek et al., 2012). Tools for editing videos vary across methods of filming. If completed with a smartphone, it is likely that videos may be edited and finalized within that same device. If another type of camera is utilized, it may be necessary to import videos to a computer and utilize editing software to produce the video model.

Implementation

The research on the frequency with which the learner should view the edited video model is somewhat ambiguous. Whereas some researchers recommend that videos should be viewed once per day, others suggest that videos may be viewed less frequently (Bellini & McConnell, 2010). Ultimately, the intensity with which video models are viewed by the learner should be determined through data-based decision-making. Interventionists may initially consider more frequent viewing of videos, with fading of intervention intensity dependent upon change in the learner's demonstration of the target social skill. Interventionists may also consider timing of viewing video models when implementing the intervention, with some researchers suggesting viewing video models immediately prior to the time when the target social skill is expected to be needed or utilized (e.g., Plavnick, 2012).

In addition to elements of frequency and timing, the physical location of the video modeling intervention should be carefully selected. The viewing environment should provide minimal distractions, with Bellini and McConnell suggesting that the interventionist should provide limited verbal interactions before, during, and following viewing of the video. In addition to decreasing environmental distractions, some learners may benefit from the addition of motivational strategies for attending to videos. For example, Charlop-Christy et al. (2000) provided praise to learners for attending to a video model, and Tetreault and Lerman (2010) provided learners with a preferred edible contingent upon attention to the video.

Intervention Evaluation

Data collection should continue during intervention as prior to intervention. That is, data collection should occur with a similar frequency and methodology, allowing for comparison of social skill demonstration prior to and following implementation of the video modeling intervention. In addition to collecting data on the social skill, Collier-Meek et al. (2012) recommend that data be collected regarding fidelity to intervention procedures, allowing the interventionist to be confident that any changes in behavior observed are related to implementation of the intervention. If an interventionist determines that the video modeling intervention is not being implemented as intended (e.g., video not being reviewed on the identified schedule), retraining or modification of intervention procedures should occur. If the interventionist is confident that the intervention has been implemented as intended, they may review data to determine whether a functional relation between the intervention and the learner's social skill use is present. Data should be regularly reviewed, such that adaptations to intervention may be made as necessary (e.g., increasing/decreasing the frequency with which the video model is viewed, addition of additional intervention procedures targeting the skill).

Practical Case Example

Starla is 15 years old with a diagnosis of ASD. Starla currently receives clinically based services to address social concerns. Starla attends individual sessions with a psychologist on a weekly basis. Starla has well-developed basic social skills, but struggles with more complex social interactions that are required to interact with her high school-age peers. Starla has expressed an interest in refining text messaging skills as a means of communicating with peers, as she indicates that she typically feels more confident in communicating with peers through this medium. However, Starla expressed that she often feels anxious when someone sends her a text message. More specifically, she indicated that she often takes a long time to determine an appropriate response to a peer, and that she is worried her peers will think that she is ignoring them or uninterested in texting with them. As such, Starla indicated that she would like to refine strategies for responding to peers via text.

The psychologist working with Starla first aimed to develop steps to responding to texts and a list of generic responses that would indicate interest in the conversation, yet also provide Starla with additional time to identify what she finds to be a meaningful response to the text. The psychologist then presented these responses to Starla for input regarding the social validity of potential responses. Starla indicated that the responses seemed like they would be okay to use with peers.

Next, the psychologist developed several video models that demonstrated use of the responding skill. Each video depicted the psychologist receiving a text message. The psychologist then verbally stated "I'm not sure how to respond to this now, but I can acknowledge the text and show interest." Following, the psychologist modeled texting responses such as "cool, let me think about it," and "gimme just a minute." A total of five different possible responses were modeled. After the videos were created, Starla and the psychologist watched the video models together and critiqued skill use. Starla was then encouraged to think of other ways that she might be able to respond to a peer to indicate interest and a need for more time for a thoughtful response. Starla then practiced these responses with the psychologist, after which she was encouraged to use this skill with peers during the week and keep track of how she did.

During their meeting the following week, Starla reported that she had used the practiced responses frequently throughout the week and that she felt less anxious about responding to peers immediately while doing so. Starla also expressed that though the response was effective, that she was repeating the same response too frequently. As such, Starla and the psychologist worked to brainstorm additional possible responses to peers' text messages. In subsequent meetings, Starla indicated that the strategy had been effective and that she was more confident in her relationships with peers.

Conclusion

VM and VSM have been used for decades to promote the acquisition and performance of social behavior in individuals with ASD. Although both are equally effective, practitioners are encouraged to consider this strategy for younger children as it appears more effective for this age group than for adolescents. Additionally, because these strategies require specific technology (e.g., camera, display device, editing software) and relevant technological skills (e.g., video editing) to implement, they may not be readily accessible to all; however, their general effectiveness and identification as an evidence-based strategy make them an appealing strategy, particularly because they can be tailored to a client's idiosyncratic needs.

References

Bandura, A. (1965). Influence of models' reinforcement contingencies on the acquisition of imitative responses. *Journal of Personality and Social Psychology, 1*, 589–595.

Bandura, A., & McClelland, D. C. (1977). *Social learning theory* (Vol. 1). Prentice Hall.

Bellini, S., & Akullian, J. (2007). A meta-analysis of video modeling and video self-modeling interventions for children and adolescents with autism spectrum disorders. *Exceptional Children, 73*, 264–287.

Bellini, S., & McConnell, L. L. (2010). Strength-based educational programming for students with autism spectrum disorders: A case for video self-modeling. *Preventing School Failure: Alternative Education for Children and Youth, 54*, 220–227.

Charlop, M. H., & Milstein, J. P. (1989). Teaching autistic children conversational speech using video modeling. *Journal of Applied Behavior Analysis, 22*, 275–285.

Charlop-Christy, M. H., Le, L., & Freeman, K. A. (2000). A comparison of video modeling with in vivo modeling for teaching children with autism. *Journal of Autism and Developmental Disorders, 30*, 537–552.

Collier-Meek, M. A., Fallon, L. M., Johnson, A. H., Sanetti, L. M., & Delcampo, M. A. (2012). Constructing self-modeling videos: Procedures and technology. *Psychology in the Schools, 49*, 3–14.

Cooper, J. O., Heron, T. E., & Heward, W. L. (2020). *Applied behavior analysis*. Pearson.

Dowrick, P. W. (1999). A review of self modeling and related interventions. *Applied and Preventive Psychology, 8*, 23–39.

Gresham, F. M. (2001). Assessment of social skills in children and adolescents. In J. Andrews, D. Saklofske, & H. Janzen (Eds.), *Handbook of psychoeducational assessment: Ability, achievement, and behavior in children* (pp. 326–326). Academic.

Haring, T. G., Kennedy, C. H., Adams, M. J., & Pitts-Conway, V. (1987). Teaching generalization of purchasing skills across community settings to autistic youth using videotape modeling. *Journal of Applied Behavior Analysis, 20*, 89–96.

Hitchcock, C. H., Dowrick, P. W., & Prater, M. A. (2003). Video self-modeling intervention in school-based settings: A review. *Remedial and Special Education, 24*, 36–45.

Lee, S. Y., Lo, Y. Y., & Lo, Y. (2017). Teaching functional play skills to a young child with autism spectrum disorder through video self-modeling. *Journal of Autism and Developmental Disorders, 47*(8), 2295–2306.

McCoy, K., & Hermansen, E. (2007). Video modeling for individuals with autism: A review of model types and effects. *Education and Treatment of Children, 30*, 183–213.

Miltenberger, C. A., & Charlop, M. H. (2015). The comparative effectiveness of portable video modeling vs. traditional video modeling interventions with children with autism spectrum disorders. *Journal of Developmental and Physical Disabilities, 27*, 341–358.

Plavnick, J. B. (2012). A practical strategy for teaching a child with autism to attend to and imitate a portable video model. *Research & Practice for Persons with Severe Disabilities, 37*, 263–270.

Qi, C. H., Barton, E. E., Collier, M., & Lin, Y. L. (2018). A systematic review of single-case research studies on using video modeling interventions to improve social communication skills for individuals with autism spectrum disorder. *Focus on Autism and Other Developmental Disabilities, 33*, 249–257.

Radley, K. C., Dart, E. H., Brennan, K. J., Helbig, K. A., Lehman, E. L., Silberman, M., & Mendanhall, K. (2020). Social skills teaching for individuals with autism spectrum disorder: A systematic review. *Advances in Neurodevelopmental Disorders, 4*, 215–226.

Sanetti, L. M. H., Collier-Meek, M. A., Long, A. C., Byron, J., & Kratochwill, T. R. (2015). Increasing teacher treatment integrity of behavior support plans through consultation and implementation planning. *Journal of School Psychology, 53*, 209–229.

Sheridan, S. M., Knoche, L. L., Edwards, C. P., Bovaird, J. A., & Kupzyk, K. A. (2010). Parent engagement and school readiness: Effects of the Getting Ready intervention on preschool children's social–emotional competencies. *Early Education and Development, 21*, 125–156.

Skinner, B. F. (1963). Operant behavior. *American Psychologist, 18*, 503–515.

Stokes, T. F., & Baer, D. M. (1977). An implicit technology of generalization. *Journal of Applied Behavior Analysis, 10*, 349–367.

Tetreault, A. S., & Lerman, D. C. (2010). Teaching social skills to children with autism using point-of-view video modeling. *Education and Treatment of Children, 33*, 395–419.

Wang, S. Y., Cui, Y., & Parrila, R. (2011). Examining the effectiveness of peer-mediated and video-modeling social skills interventions for children with autism spectrum disorders: A meta-analysis in single-case research using HLM. *Research in Autism Spectrum Disorders, 5*, 562–569.

Chapter 4
Behavioral Skills Training

Behavioral Skills Training (BST) is a multi-component instructional method that is used to promote the acquisition of new skills and behaviors. For this reason, BST should be strongly considered when attempting to address social skill acquisition deficits. One of the first uses of the term behavioral skills training appears in a doctoral dissertation examining its effect, in combination with systematic desensitization, on teachers' anxiety during instruction (Dollar, 1972). Since then, BST has been used in a vast number of studies to promote skill acquisition across a wide variety of target skills and populations. One of its most popular uses is to teach clinic and school staff members to implement behavioral treatment programs. For example, Sarokoff and Sturmey (2004) used BST to teach clinical staff members how to implement a discrete trial teaching program and Hogan et al. (2015) used it to teach school staff members how to implement students' behavior intervention plans.

BST has also been used to teach other skills including adaptive behavior and safety skills, social behavior and communication, and parent implementation of treatment programs. For example, Miltenberger (2008) and Johnson et al. (2006) used BST to teach gun safety and abduction-prevention behaviors to young children, respectively. Miles and Wilder (2009) used BST to teach parents to implement a behavioral treatment program to address noncompliance in children. Tai and Miltenberger (2017) used BST to teach safe tackling skills to children in a youth football league. Seiverling et al. (2012) used BST to teach parents to address food selectivity exhibited by their children. Finally, Thomas et al. (2016) used BST to teach an 11-year-old boy with ASD five skateboarding skills. Although these are just a small sample of the available literature supporting BST as an effective instructional method, these studies provide a view of the scope of skills it has been used to teach.

K. C Radley, E. H. Dart, *Social Skills Teaching for Individuals with Autism*,
Springer Series on Child and Family Studies,
https://doi.org/10.1007/978-3-030-91665-7_4

Components of BST

Regardless of the specific skills being taught through a BST model or the population of learners being targeted, BST is always composed of the following four components, which are typically implemented in sequence: instruction, modeling, rehearsal, and feedback. Each component is described in fuller detail below.

Instruction Instruction can take many forms but serves the purpose of communicating to the learner the information to be learned. In BST, the instructional component serves as the mechanism through which the target behavior is described in sufficient detail so that learners understand what is expected of them. Instruction can vary along a number of dimensions including duration and modality. For example, Parsons and Reid (1995) provided clinical supervisors with "4 hours of classroom training" (p. 319) that included instruction and a discussion of printed handouts describing the skill acquisition program they were responsible for overseeing. Miltenberger et al. (2004) used the first part of a 15–20 min BST session with their child participants to discuss "the dangers of playing with guns and [describe] three safety skills" (p. 514). Rosales et al. (2009) trained adults to use a picture exchange communication system with their clients by first having them watch a 26-min instructional video on the system and reviewing a checklist of the requisite skills. As these selected examples demonstrate, the nature of instruction can vary.

When BST is used for social skills instruction, it is common to provide not only a verbal description of the skill to be taught but also a rationale for why it is being taught and descriptions of situations in which the skill should be used. Dogan et al. (2017) trained parents of children with ASD to implement a BST program to teach their children two social skills, joining a conversation and asking for help. For the instructional component, parents were expected to introduce each skill and provide a rationale for why it is important, describe the specific steps of the skill, allow the learner to ask any questions about the skill, and provide the learner an opportunity to recite the steps of the skill to ensure understanding. These procedures represent typical practice when using BST to teach social skills; however, the specific instructional steps can vary based on the needs of the learner and the skills being taught. As mentioned previously, the instructional component of BST is typically the first, and often the briefest component. Once a learner has received the instructional knowledge they advance to the modeling portion of the training paradigm.

Modeling As discussed in the previous chapter, modeling involves demonstrating the skill or behavior to be taught and capitalizes on the idea of observational learning to drive treatment effects. Within BST, modeling serves the purpose of reinforcing the information provided during the instructional component, allowing the learner to see the information come to life without yet requiring them to demonstrate the skill themselves. In the broader BST literature, modeling can take many forms. For example, to teach the three gun safety behaviors to children, Miltenberger et al. (2004) had the child participants watch an adult trainer find an actual handgun in a room before exhibiting the safety behaviors. Thomas et al.' (2016) study using

BST to teach skateboarding skills had the trainer model the skill three times in front of the participant before moving onto the rehearsal component. It is important that the individual responsible for modeling the skill being taught has mastered it themselves. Otherwise, they may provide an incorrect or inappropriate model, leading to confusion or delays in appropriate skill acquisition.

When using BST to teach social skills to individuals with ASD, the modeling component generally takes one of two forms. The first is to have the individual responsible for implementing BST model the social skill. The second is to provide a VM or VSM of the skill occurring. Both have been used effectively for this purpose. Dogan et al.' (2017) parent implemented BST program had parents announce that they would demonstrate the social skill, describe a scenario in which the skill would be used, demonstrate the skill within the context of the scenario, and check again to see if the learner had any questions. On the other hand, Radley et al. (2015) evaluation of the Superheroes Social Skills program, which uses a BST package to promote skill acquisition, used a video model of children exhibiting the skills being taught. Video models are more commonly associated with manualized curricula based on a BST framework, as will be discussed in Chap. 8. Once the social skill has been modeled for the learner, they are then given the opportunity to practice, or rehearse, the newly learned skill.

Rehearsal Rehearsal is the act of engaging in a behavior one or more times in order to become more accurate or increase the fluency with which you can exhibit it. Within BST, the rehearsal component provides the learner their first opportunity to demonstrate the skill being taught as well as providing the instructor their first opportunity to evaluate the learner's performance of the skill. Depending on the specifics of the BST package and the target skill, rehearsal may look a little different. That is, rehearsal of a behavior exhibited over a duration of time (e.g., academic engagement) might have the learner engage in the behavior for a brief but continuous period. For example, Hogan et al.' (2015) evaluation of BST to promote behavior plan implementation by school staff members had them implementing the behavior plans over a 10-min period. A more discrete skill, like abduction-prevention behaviors, might be rehearsed once or one in repetition. For example, Johnson et al. (2006) had children exhibit abduction-prevention behaviors within a roleplay environment where the trainers attempted to lure them away with one of four different lures. Rehearsal activities can occur in either naturalistic or contrived (i.e., roleplay) settings. The choice of either depends largely on whether a naturalistic setting is available for rehearsal. That is, it may be more feasible to rehearse skateboarding skills in a naturalistic setting than it is to rehearse abduction-prevention behaviors simply because the opportunities to respond to the former are much greater than those of the latter.

When using BST to teach social skills, rehearsal is often conducted in a contrived setting. In fact, it is often the instructor or teacher implementing BST who is responsible for creating a situation in which a particular social skill should be used. Dogan et al. (2017) had parents describe a social scenario to their child before providing them with a prompt to rehearse one of the two social skills they were targeting through BST. Because social skills are often short, discrete behaviors, their rehearsal may be brief, requiring only a quick hypothetical scenario before a prompt is given to the learner to exhibit the skill. For example, to have a learner rehearse the social skill of requesting assistance, a teacher using BST may tell them to pretend they are in a grocery store and want to find the pizza sauce. The teacher can then describe themselves as an employee of the grocery store and prompt the learner to request assistance from them to find the pizza sauce. In this way, the teacher has given the learner one opportunity to rehearse the social skill of requesting assistance. This can be repeated multiple times and using as many exemplar scenarios as the teacher can conjure. Once the learner has rehearsed the skill, the final step in BST is to provide them with feedback on their performance.

Feedback Feedback, or performance feedback, is the process of conveying to an individual how their behavior compared to the criterion for performance of that skill. Performance feedback has been used to increase intervention agents' adherence to treatment protocols (e.g., Noell et al., 2005). Within BST, the feedback component provides the learner the opportunity to receive information about what steps of the skill were performed accurately and which were not. Unlike the feedback individuals may receive about their behavior in naturalistic settings (e.g., the peer-review process), the feedback component in BST is delivered immediately following rehearsal of the skill. The close temporal proximity between the two increases the likelihood that behavioral change will occur as a result of the feedback. However, in order to provide a learner with this information, it is necessary to set a criterion for performance. When teaching social behavior, operational definitions and tasks analyses (discussed in Chap. 2) serve as the criteria for performance and can be used to provide structured and objective feedback to a learner. In fact, it is not uncommon for a teacher to go step by step through a skill's task analysis and convey to the learner whether each step was exhibited accurately or not. In giving feedback, teachers can also provide learners with reminders about what they should have done differently as well as reinforcement (e.g., praise) for what they did correctly. It is important that learners receive feedback after every time the skill is rehearsed, even if the feedback is praise for exhibiting the skill with 100% accuracy.

The BST Cycle Now that the essential components of BST have been described, you may be wondering what happens after feedback is delivered to an individual following their rehearsal of the social skill. In most cases, unless they exhibited the skill with perfect accuracy, the BST process is recycled, although not necessarily beginning again with instruction. Instead, learners are usually given another opportunity to rehearse immediately after receiving feedback from their most recent rehearsal. This rehearsal-feedback cycle can then continue until the learner exhibits the behavior with 100% accuracy at which point the BST process is considered complete. Setting a mastery criterion in this way ensures that the teaching process continues until the teacher can be confident that the learner's responding is independent and no longer reliant on prompts or additional feedback.

Empirical Basis of BST

Since first described in the literature, BST has received substantial support as a procedure for promoting social skill acquisition and use. In considering the literature, support can be found for each of the individual elements with BST (i.e., instruction, modeling, rehearsal, feedback), as well as BST as a package of intervention elements. A brief review of the support for these elements for social skills teaching, combined and separately, is described below.

Instruction

Whereas some elements of BST are frequently evaluated in isolation from other social skills teaching strategies, instruction is rarely implemented as a stand-alone social skills teaching strategy for learners with ASD. Instead, didactic instruction may more commonly be found in social skills teaching strategies that are not targeted toward a particular individual or group of students (e.g., classwide social skills lesson). In one example of instruction being relied upon as the primary mechanism of change, Russo-Ponsaran et al. (2016) utilized didactic instruction to promote recognition of facial emotions in children and adolescents with ASD. Instruction in the study consisted of participants viewing videos of facial emotions while a voice over described salient features of the face that indicate a particular emotion. Researchers found that participation in the intervention resulted in increased accuracy and speed of identification of emotions by participants with ASD.

In another example, Bradley (2019) provided rules to children with ASD as a means of promoting social skill use. During training with instructions, the researcher described the importance of using the target skill (i.e., saying thank you following compliments). Checks for knowledge were also implemented, with the researcher asking participants what should be said following a compliment from someone else. Finally, the researcher trained other scenarios in which the use of thank you would be warranted, such as when someone helps or gives something to you. Results presented indicate that use of rules was effective in increasing social skill use of participants included in the study. The results presented by Bradley suggest that a relatively low intensity intervention (i.e., describing social skill use rules) may be sufficient to increase use of some social skills. In other cases, however, more comprehensive teaching strategies may be warranted (e.g., Gresham et al., 2001).

Modeling

Of the individual BST elements, modeling is perhaps implemented most frequently as a stand-alone intervention. This often takes the form of video modeling (see Chap. 3), with an individual viewing video recorded demonstrations of target social skills. In vivo modeling can be implemented in isolation as well, with Charlop-Christy et al. (2000) providing an example of the utility of this strategy. Skills addressed within the intervention included skills such as identifying emotions in others and playing cooperative games. Results of the study suggested that video modeling resulted in more rapid acquisition of the target skills; however, skills addressed using in vivo modeling alone also demonstrated improvement. Subsequent systematic replications have documented the efficacy of both in vivo and video models in resulting in acquisition and use of skills (e.g., Gena et al., 2005; Wilson, 2013).

Peers may also serve as models to promote social skill use. Harper et al. (2008) trained six elementary-age students to engage in social interaction skills, indicating that these skills could be used with two peers with ASD. Prior to recess periods, the students were prompted to use the skills with their peers with ASD during play. Following training, peers with ASD were observed to increase the frequency of use of the same skills modeled by the other students, specifically, gaining attention, initiating play, and turn-taking. Use of modeling as done by Harper et al. (2008) may also confer additional benefits not explicitly evaluated as part of the study, as peers who interact and are able to model skill use across a variety of contexts—promoting maintenance and generalization of skills.

Rehearsal

Similar to instruction, rehearsal is seldom used in isolation of other elements of BST. Interventions provided to individuals with ASD rarely provide *only* opportunities to respond or rehearse a skill, instead typically providing some other support (e.g., description of the skill to rehearse) in conjunction with the opportunity to rehearse the skill. It is possible to conceptualize peer-mediated interventions, described in Chap. 6, as representing rehearsal interventions for the learner with ASD. Within these interventions, instruction may be provided to peers in strategies for interacting with learners with ASD—who then go and utilize the newly learned interactional skills in realistic settings (i.e., with the learner with ASD). The learner with ASD does not contact any direct instruction, modeling, or feedback; instead, they only contact increased opportunities to respond or rehearse social interactions. An example of an intervention that provides only rehearsal to the learner with ASD can be found in Kohler et al. (2007), who found such an intervention to result in increased peer-directed overtures of a learner with ASD.

For learners who demonstrate acquisition or performance deficits, it is unlikely that an intervention that only provides increased opportunities to respond would be sufficient. That is, such an intervention would not meet the instructional needs of the learner. Gresham (1998) suggests that some learners may present with fluency deficits, which may be the result of insufficient opportunities to practice or rehearse a particular skill. It is only for this type of deficit that rehearsal-only interventions may be appropriate.

Feedback

Feedback-only interventions entail strategies in which a learner receives feedback on a skill already in their repertoire. Tagavi et al. (2020) provide an example of a feedback-only intervention to address social communication in a study including three adults with ASD. Instead of providing instruction in social communication skills, the intervention entailed participants engaging in a conversation while being filmed, and then viewing this recording while completing a self-evaluation of conversational fluidity. This intervention, in which feedback on skill use was obtained through self-evaluation, was found to increase the duration of fluid conversation across all participants. Other interventions have provided feedback face-to-face (e.g., Yamamoto & Isawa, 2020) to similar effect.

Behavioral Skills Training

As reviewed above, the individual components within BST may be implemented in isolation. However, interventions including one component of BST tend to incorporate multiple or all indicated elements. Several researchers have conducted component analyses of BST, with most indicating that the combined implementation of BST elements is typically more effective than implementation of any one component in isolation (e.g., Drifke et al., 2017). Regarding BST for social skills, Kornacki et al. (2013) failed to identify a single component of BST that was associated with the greatest level of change in social skill use, with the authors suggesting that attempting to implement a single component in isolation may ultimately be a less efficient strategy than implementing BST as a package.

Overall, BST represents one of the most frequently implemented social skills teaching strategies (Radley et al., 2020). In a meta-analysis of BST for learners with ASD, Roth et al. (2014) found BST to produce moderate effects, with interventions targeting outcomes such as initiating conversations, turn taking, answering questions, and joining in group activities. Watkins et al. (2017), in a meta-analysis of school-based interventions for adolescents with ASD, also found BST to be supported as an effective intervention for addressing social skills.

The studies included in reviews and meta-analyses of BST have addressed a wide range of social skills, including conversation skills, responding to peers, greetings, giving compliments, taking turns, abduction prevention, and modulation of nonverbal behaviors (e.g., Leaf et al., 2016). In one example of using BST for social skills teaching, Nuernberger et al. (2013) taught vocal and non-vocal conversation skills to young adults with ASD. Following teaching, participants demonstrated improvements in accuracy of skill use that was maintained over time. Ryan et al. (2019) found conversation skills to improve following BST, again with changes in skill use being maintained over time.

Although researchers and practitioners directly implement BST to teach social skills, other studies have evaluated BST as implemented by other stakeholders. As previously described, Dogan et al. (2017) used parent-implemented BST to promote joining in a conversation and asking for help in children with ASD—finding the procedures to result in rapid acquisition of the target skills. Similarly, Hassan et al. (2018) found that parent-implemented BST was effective in increasing their children's use of social skills. However, parents in Hassan et al.'s study did require additional, in situ supports that were not provided by Dogan et al. in order to implement BST with integrity—with accuracy of skill use by children with ASD increasing as parents implemented BST with a greater degree of integrity.

In addition to parents (e.g., Stewart et al., 2007), peers have also been trained to effectively implement BST for social skills. Beaulieu et al. (2014) designed an intervention for a college-age individual who indicated a desire to learn to maintain conversations. Peers consisted of same-age college students, who the individual with ASD knew were assisting with intervention implementation. Results indicated that implementation of BST resulted in decreased interrupting and increased questioning during conversations with peers. Further emphasizing the meaningfulness of change, changes in social communication were observed during conversation with generalized peers following termination of intervention procedures.

Taken together, the body of literature supporting BST as a means of promoting social behavior is strong. Researchers have found BST to be effective across implementers (e.g., researchers, parents, peers). Studies have included participants of varying ages from elementary (e.g., Leaf et al., 2009) to college (e.g., Beaulieu et al., 2014). BST has also been found to be effective when implemented individually (e.g., Kassardjian et al., 2013) or in groups (Dotson et al., 2010). Furthermore, evidence supports use of BST for social skills training for individuals with (e.g., Ng et al., 2016) and without (e.g., Peters et al., 2016) co-morbid intellectual disability. Taken together, the extant evidence supports use of BST for social skills teaching with individuals with ASD.

Other Practical Considerations

DiGennaro Reed et al. (2018) provide a concise summary of BST as well as a practical guide to create video models to use during the modeling component. Although geared toward teacher implementation of interventions within a classroom setting, several important considerations are raised that may be useful to consider in designing BST programs for social skill instruction with individuals with ASD. First, they recommend monitoring the progress of learners once BST is completed to ensure that skill acquisition maintains in the absence of additional teaching. As mentioned in Chap. 2, social skill accuracy data can be collected during both the acquisition process and the performance process. Although BST is designed to remediate acquisition deficits, it is not safe to assume the work is done after skill acquisition is complete. In fact, you may find that what was once an acquisition deficit is now a performance deficit, requiring additional environmental modifications to address now that the skill has been learned. Continuous monitoring of skill use can aid in this type of decision-making.

Relatedly, DiGenarro and colleagues recommend engaging in directed rehearsal with the learner. Directed rehearsal is similar to rehearsal within the BST process except it is focused on only those steps that were exhibited incorrectly during a naturalistic observation. That is, the teacher may, during the progress monitoring process, find that a learner is exhibiting five out of the six steps for initiating a conversation correctly while on the playground at school. Directed rehearsal would have the teacher meet with the learner at another time and provide specific feedback about the incorrect step before asking them to rehearse the full skill several times with them. In this way, directed rehearsal bridges the gap between a contrived BST environment and the naturalistic environment in which the skill is expected to be used.

Finally, to support continued skill performance following acquisition, DiGennaro Reed et al. (2018) recommend establishing a contingency of reinforcement for skill use in the target environment. Although social skills often contact sources of reinforcement naturally (e.g., reduction in task aversiveness after requesting assistance, social reinforcement during conversation), an individual with no learning history of contacting these contingencies may need additional support at first. Establishing a new contingency (e.g., differential reinforcement of appropriate behavior; DRA, see Chap. 10) with salient discriminative stimuli may be a good place to begin before engaging in efforts to transfer stimulus control to the natural environment.

Practical Case Example

Imagine you are leading a social skills group in a school-based setting that uses behavioral skills training as its primary treatment modality. In this group, which meets for 30 min once each week, a different social behavior is targeted. Through interviews with the student participants, their classroom teachers, and their caregivers, you have compiled a list of ten social skills that you will be teaching across a 10-week period. You have decided to use BST as your teaching strategy because it works well in a group setting and is one of the most effective ways to remediate acquisition deficits. Let us look at how one of the skills, terminating a conversation, might be addressed in this format.

First, didactic instruction would begin with an introduction to the skill, why it might be important, and what it looks like. You might say "Today we are going to talk about ending conversations. When we are talking to others we sometimes need to find a way to tell them we are finished talking or that we need to leave. To do that, it might be best to first think of a reason for why you are ending the conversation, wait for a pause or break in the conversation, provide the reason to your conversational partner, and say goodbye." This example accomplishes the goal of introducing the skill, providing some context for its social importance, and briefly describing how one might go about exhibiting the skill. Next, you would model the skill in front of the group participants. To accomplish this, it might be best to recruit one of the group members to hold a conversation with you and then demonstrate how you terminate the conversation appropriately. While doing so, it would also be beneficial to verbalize each of the steps of the skill as they occur or shortly after (e.g., "See how I waited for a pause in the conversation instead of interrupting?"). You may choose to repeat the modeling of the skill or recruit a different group member to engage in a different model exercise with you to provide participants additional exemplars. Next, it is time to allow the group members to practice or roleplay the skill themselves. It might be best to have one of the group members rehearse the skill with you at a time, allowing the others another opportunity to observe the skill being modeled. In doing so, you would hold a conversation with a group member until they attempt to terminate the conversation using the steps provided to them during the instruction and modeling phase. Immediately after a group member attempts to terminate the conversation with you, you would provide specific feedback regarding the steps of the skill they implemented correctly and those they implemented incorrectly. For example, you might say "That was great! I like how you told me your ride was here and you had to leave but remember next time to wait until there is a pause in the conversation so we don't interrupt when someone else is speaking." Give each group member the chance to practice the skill in this way with you while the others observe until each group member has exhibited the skill with 100% accuracy. Then, you may choose to give overall feedback to the group related to common mistakes or things everyone did well. Finally, you may choose to have the group members rehearse the skill with each other or you may choose to return to the instructional phase if it appears additional instruction is necessary.

Conclusion

To summarize, BST is an evidence-based strategy that has been used for decades to teach new behaviors to individuals, including social skills to individuals with ASD. Its four relatively simple components of instruction, modeling, rehearsal, and feedback provide a concrete paradigm to promote skill acquisition while remaining flexible enough in its implementation to meet the needs of a wide range of learners. Those faced with remediated social skill acquisition deficits in individuals with ASD are encouraged to incorporate BST into their treatment package to drive effective and efficient change.

References

Beaulieu, L., Hanley, G. P., & Santiago, J. L. (2014). Improving the conversational skills of a college student with peer-mediated behavioral skills training. *The Analysis of Verbal Behavior, 30*(1), 48–53.

Bradley, R. L. (2019). *Rule-governed behavior: Teaching essential school readiness skills via rule-following to children with autism.* Unpublished doctoral dissertation, Louisiana State University.

Charlop-Christy, M. H., Le, L., & Freeman, K. A. (2000). A comparison of video modeling with in vivo modeling for teaching children with autism. *Journal of Autism and Developmental Disorders, 30*, 537–552.

DiGennaro Reed, F. D., Blackman, A. L., Erath, T. G., Brand, D., & Novak, M. D. (2018). Guidelines for using behavioral skills training to provide teacher support. *Teaching Exceptional Children, 50*, 373–380.

Dogan, R. K., King, M. L., Fischetti, A. T., Lake, C. M., Mathews, T. L., & Warzak, W. J. (2017). Parent-implemented behavioral skills training of social skills. *Journal of Applied Behavior Analysis, 50*, 805–818.

Dollar, B. L. (1972). *The effects of desensitization and behavioral skills training on situational teaching anxiety.* Doctoral dissertation, ProQuest Information & Learning.

Dotson, W. H., Leaf, J. B., Sheldon, J. B., & Sherman, J. A. (2010). Group teaching of conversational skills to adolescents on the autism spectrum. *Research in Autism Spectrum Disorders, 4*, 199–209.

Drifke, M. A., Tiger, J. H., & Wierzba, B. C. (2017). Using behavioral skills training to teach parents to implement three-step prompting: A component analysis and generalization assessment. *Learning and Motivation, 57*, 1–14.

Gena, A., Couloura, S., & Kymissis, E. (2005). Modifying the affective behavior of preschoolers with autism using in-vivo or video modeling and reinforcement contingencies. *Journal of Autism and Developmental Disorders, 35*, 545–556.

Gresham, F. M. (1998). Social skills training: Should we raze, remodel, or rebuild? *Behavioral Disorders, 24*, 19–25.

Gresham, F. M., Sugai, G., & Horner, R. H. (2001). Interpreting outcomes of social skills training for students with high-incidence disabilities. *Exceptional Children, 67*, 331–344.

Harper, C. B., Symon, J. B., & Frea, W. D. (2008). Recess is time-in: Using peers to improve social skills of children with autism. *Journal of Autism and Developmental Disorders, 38*, 815–826.

Hassan, M., Simpson, A., Danaher, K., Haesen, J., Makela, T., & Thomson, K. (2018). An evaluation of behavioral skills training for teaching caregivers how to support social skill development in their child with autism spectrum disorder. *Journal of Autism and Developmental Disorders, 48*, 1957–1970.

Hogan, A., Knez, N., & Kahng, S. (2015). Evaluating the use of behavioral skills training to improve school staffs' implementation of behavior intervention plans. *Journal of Behavioral Education, 24*, 242–254.

Johnson, B. M., Miltenberger, R. G., Knudson, P., Egemo-Helm, K., Kelso, P., Jostad, C., & Langley, L. (2006). A preliminary evaluation of two behavioral skills training procedures for teaching abduction-prevention skills to schoolchildren. *Journal of Applied Behavior Analysis, 39*, 25–34.

Kassardjian, A., Rudrud, E., Taubman, M., Leaf, J. B., Edwards, A., Schulze, K., et al. (2013). Utilizing teaching interactions to facilitate social skills in the natural environment. *Education and Training in Autism and Developmental Disabilities, 48*, 245–257.

Kohler, F. W., Greteman, C., Raschke, D., & Highnam, C. (2007). Using a buddy skills package to increase the social interactions between a preschooler with autism and her peers. *Topics in Early Childhood Special Education, 27*, 155–163.

Kornacki, L. T., Ringdahl, J. E., Sjostrom, A., & Nuernberger, J. E. (2013). A component analysis of a behavioral skills training package used to teach conversation skills to young adults with autism spectrum and other developmental disorders. *Research in Autism Spectrum Disorders, 7*, 1370–1376.

Leaf, J. B., Leaf, R., McEachin, J., Taubman, M., Ala'i-Rosales, S., Ross, R. K., et al. (2016). Applied behavior analysis is a science and, therefore, progressive. *Journal of Autism and Developmental Disorders, 46*, 720–731.

Leaf, J. B., Taubman, M., Bloomfield, S., Palos-Rafuse, L., Leaf, R., McEachin, J., & Oppenheim, M. L. (2009). Increasing social skills and pro-social behavior for three children diagnosed with autism through the use of a teaching package. *Research in Autism Spectrum Disorders, 3*, 275–289.

Miles, N. I., & Wilder, D. A. (2009). The effects of behavioral skills training on caregiver implementation of guided compliance. *Journal of Applied Behavior Analysis, 42*, 405–410.

Miltenberger, R. G. (2008). Teaching safety skills to children: Prevention of firearm injury as an exemplar of best practice in assessment, training, and generalization of safety skills. *Behavior Analysis in Practice, 1*, 30–36.

Miltenberger, R. G., Flessner, C., Gatheridge, B., Johnson, B., Satterlund, M., & Egemo, K. (2004). Evaluation of behavioral skills training to prevent gun play in children. *Journal of Applied Behavior Analysis, 37*, 513–516.

Ng, A. H. S., Schulze, K., Rudrud, E., & Leaf, J. B. (2016). Using the teaching interactions procedure to teach social skills to children with autism and intellectual disability. *American Journal on Intellectual and Developmental Disabilities, 121*, 501–519.

Noell, G. H., Witt, J. C., Slider, N. J., Connell, J. E., Gatti, S. L., Williams, K. L., et al. (2005). Treatment implementation following behavioral consultation in schools: A comparison of three follow-up strategies. *School Psychology Review, 34*, 87–106.

Nuernberger, J. E., Ringdahl, J. E., Vargo, K. K., Crumpecker, A. C., & Gunnarsson, K. F. (2013). Using a behavioral skills training package to teach conversation skills to young adults with autism spectrum disorders. *Research in Autism Spectrum Disorders, 7*, 411–417.

Parsons, M. B., & Reid, D. H. (1995). Training residential supervisors to provide feedback for maintaining staff teaching skills with people who have severe disabilities. *Journal of Applied Behavior Analysis, 28*, 317–322.

Peters, B., Tullis, C. A., & Gallagher, P. A. (2016). Effects of a group teaching interaction procedure on the social skills of students with autism spectrum disorders. *Education and Training in Autism and Developmental Disabilities, 51*, 421–433.

Radley, K. C., Dart, E. H., Brennan, K. J., Helbig, K. A., Lehman, E. L., Silberman, M., & Mendanhall, K. (2020). Social skills teaching for individuals with autism spectrum disorder: A systematic review. *Advances in Neurodevelopmental Disorders, 4*, 215–226.

Radley, K. C., Ford, W. B., McHugh, M. B., Dadakhodjaeva, K., O'Handley, R. D., Battaglia, A. A., & Lum, J. D. (2015). Brief report: Use of superheroes social skills to promote accurate social skill use in children with autism spectrum disorder. *Journal of Autism and Developmental Disorders, 45*, 3048–3054.

Rosales, R., Stone, K., & Rehfeldt, R. A. (2009). The effects of behavioral skills training on implementation of the picture exchange communication system. *Journal of Applied Behavior Analysis, 42*, 541–549.

Roth, M. E., Gillis, J. M., & Reed, F. D. D. (2014). A meta-analysis of behavioral interventions for adolescents and adults with autism spectrum disorders. *Journal of Behavioral Education, 23*, 258–286.

Russo-Ponsaran, N. M., Evans-Smith, B., Johnson, J., Russo, J., & McKown, C. (2016). Efficacy of a facial emotion training program for children and adolescents with autism spectrum disorders. *Journal of Nonverbal Behavior, 40*, 13–38.

Ryan, G., Brady, S., Holloway, J., & Lydon, H. (2019). Increasing appropriate conversation skills using a behavioral skills training package for adults with intellectual disability and autism spectrum disorder. *Journal of Intellectual Disabilities, 23*, 567–580.

Sarokoff, R. A., & Sturmey, P. (2004). The effects of behavioral skills training on staff implementation of discrete-trial teaching. *Journal of Applied Behavior Analysis, 37*, 535–538.

Seiverling, L., Williams, K., Sturmey, P., & Hart, S. (2012). Effects of behavioral skills training on parental treatment of children's food selectivity. *Journal of Applied Behavior Analysis, 45*, 197–203.

Stewart, K. K., Carr, J. E., & LeBlanc, L. A. (2007). Evaluation of family-implemented behavioral skills training for teaching social skills to a child with Asperger's disorder. *Clinical Case Studies, 6*, 252–262.

Tagavi, D., Koegel, L., Koegel, R., & Vernon, T. (2020). Improving conversational fluidity in young adults with autism spectrum disorder using a video-feedback intervention. *Journal of Positive Behavior Interventions, 23*, 245–256.

Tai, S. S., & Miltenberger, R. G. (2017). Evaluating behavioral skills training to teach safe tackling skills to youth football players. *Journal of Applied Behavior Analysis, 50*, 849–855.

Thomas, B. R., Lafasakis, M., & Spector, V. (2016). Brief report: Using behavioral skills training to teach skateboarding skills to a child with autism spectrum disorder. *Journal of Autism and Developmental Disorders, 46*, 3824–3829.

Watkins, L., O'Reilly, M., Ledbetter-Cho, K., Lang, R., Sigafoos, J., Kuhn, M., Lim, N., Gervarter, C., & Caldwell, N. (2017). A meta-analysis of school-based social interaction interventions for adolescents with autism spectrum disorder. *Review Journal of Autism and Developmental Disorders, 4*, 277–293.

Wilson, K. P. (2013). Teaching social-communication skills to preschoolers with autism: Efficacy of video versus in vivo modeling in the classroom. *Journal of Autism and Developmental Disorders, 43*, 1819–1831.

Yamamoto, S., & Isawa, S. (2020). Effects of textual prompts and feedback on social niceties of adolescents with autism spectrum disorder in a simulated workplace. *Journal of Applied Behavior Analysis, 53*, 1404–1418.

Chapter 5
Social Narratives

Social narratives are a class of evidence-based interventions used to promote social skill acquisition and encourage appropriate skill use by providing learners with a story-like narrative. These narratives often provide a description of the skill to be taught, a rationale for its use, and a wealth of contextual details for the learner to understand when and why it might be used. Unlike the previously discussed strategies (i.e., video modeling, behavioral skills training), social narratives do not involve any demonstration of the skill being performed other than the written or read depiction within the narrative itself. Social narratives may include pictures depicting models exhibiting the skill; however, unlike video models they are static and do not allow the learner to see the skill exhibited in real time. Nonetheless, social narratives have a long history of use to teach social skills to individuals with ASD.

Social narratives developed from a more specific strategy called Social Stories™ (Gray, 1998), first described by Carol Gray. Gray developed a five-part philosophy and ten criteria that underlie the Social Story™ method and are used to guide the creation of new narratives. The philosophy asks that parents and professionals working with individuals with ASD abandon their assumptions about an individual's behavior and consider social deficits as shared between two or more people. That is, Gray (1998) suggests that all parties included in a social interaction share responsibility for making it successful. Further, she encourages those working with individuals with ASD to view all perspectives as valid, not argue against someone's perception, and remain curious and hopeful about finding effective intervention strategies. With these philosophical principles in mind, we will review the ten components of a Social Story™.

First, Gray (1998) defines a Social Story™ as a narrative that "accurately describes a context, skill, achievement, or concept according to ten defining criteria." (p. 1). The ten criteria then outline the necessary elements to turn a social narrative into a Social Story™. First, Social Story™ authors are encouraged to "share accurate information using a content, format, and voice that is descriptive,

K. C Radley, E. H. Dart, *Social Skills Teaching for Individuals with Autism*,
Springer Series on Child and Family Studies,
https://doi.org/10.1007/978-3-030-91665-7_5

meaningful, and physically, socially, and emotionally safe for the audience" (p. 2). Next, authors work to gain an understanding of their audience's perspective of the social situation and identify the most critical information to be included within the story. For teaching social skills, this step will be similar to creating a task analysis (see Chap. 2). The third criterion involves the structure of the Social Story™. Specifically, each Social Story™ will contain a title that makes the topic clear, a body that provides the narrative content with contextual details, and a conclusion that summarizes what occurred and reinforces the learning objectives. The fourth criterion stipulates that the narrative is individualized to the individual learner's abilities and interests, meaning the language used is appropriate for their developmental level and the narrative context incorporates any specific interests they may have that are relevant to the social situation.

The next few criteria provide specifications about the actual writing of the narrative content. Specifically, the fifth criterion states that a Social Story™ uses only first-person (i.e., "I") or third-person language (i.e., "They"), is written in past, present, or future tense, uses a positive and patient tone, and is accurate in grammatical structure, content, and meaning. The sixth criterion requires that a Social Story™ answer relevant "WH" questions (i.e., Who, What, When, Where, and Why?) in its narrative content. That is, it should include information about the steps of the social skill (i.e., What?), the person or persons involved in the social interaction (i.e., Who?), the time and place it should be exhibited (i.e., When and Where), and the reasons for exhibiting the skill within that context (i.e., Why?). The seventh criterion specifies the two types of sentences that make up the narrative content, descriptive sentences and directive sentences. Two additional sentence types were added in a later revision to the criteria: perspective and control (Gray, 2000). Descriptive sentences provide contextual information to the learner and serve to answer the "WH" questions in a manner that is free of bias or judgment. A good example of a descriptive sentence within a Social Story™ about initiating a conversation might be "Sometimes I want to say something to my friend." The statement describes a desire to share information with a peer. Directive sentences guide or direct learner behavior by suggesting appropriate responses. A good example of a coaching sentence within a Social Story™ about initiating a conversation might be "When I want to say something to my friend I look at them and say their name." Perspective sentences describe what others might be thinking about the learner's behavior. For example: "Your friends like it when you ask them questions about themselves." Control sentences function similar to a mnemonic device by providing a narrative analogy for the learner to remember to exhibit the skill at a later time. For example: "When the fire alarm rings, think about the dinosaurs following each other out of the forest to escape the burning meteors" (Morris, 2021, p. 1). The eight criterion specifies that a Social Story™ contain at least twice as many descriptive sentences as coaching sentences.

The ninth criterion requires that Social Story™ authors present a first draft to parents, caregivers, and other key stakeholders for feedback to ensure that the content is appropriate and make any necessary edits. This process is similar to what was described in Chap. 2 when making task analyses. The tenth and final criterion is more like a short guide to editing and implementing a Social Story™, including suggestions such as Plan a Positive Introduction and Mix & Match to Build Concepts. Adhering to Gray's (1998) philosophical underpinnings and ten criteria while crafting a social narrative is necessary if the resulting product is to be identified as a Social Story™. Otherwise, it would be more appropriate to identify the product as a social narrative.

Social narratives, including Social Stories™, are frequently used to promote social skill acquisition among individuals with ASD. From a behavior analytic standpoint, social narratives function as an antecedent intervention whereby the learner is exposed to novel or less familiar social situations and appropriate reactions to those situations are described. The hope is that learners internalize the information presented in the narrative and exhibit the responses themselves in a similar social context. Therefore, social narratives are likely most appropriate to remediate social skills acquisition deficits; however, because they often describe the reinforcing consequences of appropriate social behavior, practitioners might also expect to see increases in skill performance. Next, we will review the empirical evidence supporting social narratives as an evidence-based practice.

Empirical Basis of Social Narratives

Similar to video modeling (see Chap. 3), social narratives have been identified as an established treatment by the May Institute's National Autism Center's National Standards Project in both 2009 and again in 2015. In the report, they are identified as a "story-based intervention package," but the report also notes that Social Stories™ are the most common intervention in this class. The two reports identified 21 and 15 story-based intervention studies meeting the project's inclusion criteria in 2009 and 2015, respectively, identifying the strategy as established to improve the communication and interpersonal skills of individuals with ASD. Further, there is evidence to support Social Stories™ as effective for individuals with comorbid ASD and intellectual disability (e.g., Reynhout & Carter, 2007), making them potentially effective for a wide range of clients. In addition to the National Standards Project endorsement, there have been multiple systematic reviews and meta-analyses investigating the empirical support for social narratives.

A systematic review by Qi et al. (2018) compared the extant evidence supporting Social Stories™ against the What Works Clearinghouse (WWC) single-case design research standards. They identified 22 single-case studies examining the impact of Social Stories™ on individual with ASD's social communication skills, among other outcomes. Although Social Stories™ appeared effective in reducing participants' inappropriate behavior, the authors identified questionable average treatment effects when they were used to promote social communication skills (i.e., median PND = 67%; mean PEM = 67%). Although their review did not examine potential moderators of treatment effects (e.g., age of participants, level of functioning, etc.), Qi et al. (2018) were mixed in their appraisal of whether Social Stories™ constitute an evidence-based practice depending on which analytic method was used. Specifically, when applying visual analytic methods, Social Stories™ were not considered an evidence-based strategy; however, when applying quantitative nonoverlap indices, Social Stories™ were considered an evidence-based strategy. Keep in mind that there also appeared to be large differences in the effect sizes depending on which outcome was being targeted with the smallest average effects observed for promoting social communication.

Although slightly older, Kokina and Kern (2010) conducted a meta-analysis of the Social Story™ literature, examining a large number of potential moderators to determine whether differential treatment effects were attributable to participant, setting, or target behavior variables. They identified 18 studies investigating the impact of Social Stories™ on participants' appropriate social behavior, inappropriate behavior, and adaptive behavior. The largest average effect size was identified in studies using Social Stories™ to reduce participants' inappropriate behavior (mean PND = 87%). Similar to Qi et al. (2018), Social Stories™ impact on participants' appropriate social behavior was questionable (mean PND = 56%). Other important moderators driving differential effects included the setting in which the Social Story™ was read (i.e., school setting more effective than home) and who was responsible for reading the story (i.e., having the learner read the story drove greater treatment effects than parent-, teacher-, or researcher-read stories). They also found that longer Social Stories™ (i.e., 11 or more sentences) were slightly more effective than those with 10 sentences or fewer. Finally, they found Social Stories™ most effective for individuals with ASD in the elementary grades (ages 6–11) than for those younger (ages 0–5) or older (ages 12+).

Test et al. (2011) also conducted a meta-analysis of the Social Stories™ literature, including 18 studies. Similar to the other syntheses, they found mixed evidence for the strategy (mean PND = 50%; range = 0–97%); however, they did not disaggregate the effect size by target behavior. Notably, Test et al. (2011) reported that nearly none of the studies included in their synthesis reported data to support the maintenance and generalization of treatment effects. Thus, it is currently unclear whether Social Stories™ drive lasting and generalizable change with their learners. They concluded by stating that Social Stories™ could not be considered an evidence-based practice at that time.

The literature supporting other social narrative strategies that do not meet the Social Story™ criteria is less developed. Coogle et al. (2018) describe four additional social narrative strategies frequently used with individuals with ASD including comic strips and cartoons, social scripts, SMART boards, and power cards. They describe the use of comic strips and cartoons as being very similar to Social Stories™ with the primary difference being a heavier emphasis on visual content and fewer words. This type of strategy would be more appropriate for individuals with limited verbal ability or for those unable to read. Social scripts are much more similar to Social Stories™ in that they use a narrative to describe a social situation and an appropriate response; however, they may not meet all ten of the criteria outlined by Gray (1998) to be considered a Social Story™. SMART boards do not represent a distinct intervention strategy but rather offer a novel method to present social narrative content. Coogle et al. (2018) recommend converting traditional social narratives into a digital format such as a Microsoft Powerpoint presentation and displaying using a SMART board. Unlike traditional digital projectors, SMART boards allow for touch interactivity, potentially increasing the learner's engagement with the social narrative content.

Finally, power cards are condensed versions of social narratives printed on a small card that a learner can keep with them. The cards usually include pictures or graphics related to the learner's interest and an abbreviated social narrative that is commonly formatted as a list of behaviors or expectations the learner is expected to exhibit. Rose (2020) conducted a systematic review of the power card literature and identified 12 studies investigating them as an intervention to promote social skills (n = 7) and other appropriate behaviors (n = 5) for individuals with ASD. Rose (2020) concluded that nearly all of the studies indicated positive effects on their intended outcomes, with 8 of the 12 studies producing PND values between 90 and 100% and the remaining three between 60 and 80%. Thus, although the literature base is considerably smaller, power cards appear to be a more effective intervention than Social Stories™; however, both strategies have been observed to produce desirable effects on their intended outcomes.

Guide to Practice

In reviewing the literature, Social Story and social narrative interventions often vary in the steps included to implementation. However, commonalities in intervention can be identified and should form the basis for use of the intervention strategy. These steps include, but may not be limited to (e.g., Crozier & Sileo, 2005; Swaggart et al., 1995): identification of the target behavior; operationally defining the target behavior; conducting a functional analysis; collecting baseline data; writing the social story; incorporating pictures or drawings into the story; using the social story with the learner; collecting data; and planning for maintenance and generalization.

The first step in implementing a Social Story or social narrative intervention is to identify the target social skill. A variety of means should be used to identify target skills, incorporating direct assessment (see Chap. 2) and rating scales from multiple stakeholders (e.g., teacher, caregiver, learner). In considering data collected, intervention targets should be prioritized based on the meaningfulness of the behavior to the learner. Behaviors that are highly socially and contextually valid, as well as those that may result in increased participation across environments (e.g., school, community), should be considered as important social skill targets. For challenging social behaviors, interventionists may consider selecting targets that represent the first behavior in a behavior chain or one that results in isolation of the learner (Crozier & Sileo, 2005).

Critical to any intervention, a thorough operational definition must be developed. Operational definitions should describe the occurrence of a target behavior instead of non-occurrence, passing what Lindsley (1991) described as the "Dead Man's

Test" (i.e., "if a dead man can do it, it is not behavior"). In addition to an operational definition describing the occurrence of a behavior, it should also describe the behavior in sufficient detail so that someone unfamiliar with the learner could recognize an occurrence (i.e., the Stranger Test). Put another way, an operational definition of a target skill should not rely on any prior knowledge of the observer or require the observer to make a subjective decision regarding whether a behavior meets the definition of the target behavior. For example, if the target behavior were greeting someone, one may wish to specify dimensions related to volume (e.g., sufficiently loud so that the conversation partner can hear the greeting).

Although not always implemented in research or applied settings, interventionists may consider conducting a functional analysis of the behavior. Functional data may be useful within a Social Story or social narrative intervention in that they may clarify antecedents and consequences related to the target social skill. In the case of a Social Story or social narrative, it may not be necessary to conduct a comprehensive analog functional analysis (e.g., Iwata et al., 1994). Instead, a procedure such as an ABC observation or other informal functional assessment (e.g., stakeholder interview) may be sufficient if it allows the interventionist to better conceptualize the target behavior and generate hypotheses regarding the learner's use of the behavior.

Once a target behavior has been operationally defined and variables related to that behavior identified, direct observation should be conducted to establish present levels of behavior. It is critical that the interventionist consider which dimensions of the target behavior are most critical. Potential dimensions of behavior that may be assessed via direct observation include, but are not limited to, frequency, duration, and latency. For example, a target behavior of waiting in line may best be assessed through duration—allowing the interventionist to determine how long a learner waited in line instead of just noting the occurrence of waiting (i.e., frequency of waiting in line). For other behaviors, frequency may be indicated (e.g., attempts to initiate an interaction with peers). Accurate selection of measurement dimensions will be critical to describing how useful the Social Story or social narrative was to the learner. Further, these data will be particularly useful in writing the social story, allowing the interventionist to link story content to actual levels of student behavior.

Next, the Social Story or social narrative can be written. As previously described, there is substantial variability in elements included in social narratives, with Social Stories including specific content. Using Gray and Garand's (1993) suggestions, a social story should be individualized to the learner and be relatively brief—approximately five sentences in length. A *descriptive* sentence should begin the social story, describing contextual variables (e.g., setting, peers, actions) related to use of the social skill. *Directive* sentences are then written, which provide information and directions for using the target behavior. Following, *perspective* sentences should be included which describe the thoughts, feelings, and reactions of other individuals within the environment. Finally, a Social Story includes *control* sentences. These sentences are analogies for skill use and serve as a tool for facilitating recall and use of the target skill. In writing the story, interventionists should ensure that it is written at a level that is understandable to the learner. Ideally, the story should be written to allow for flexibility (e.g., across settings, in the target behavior; Crozier & Sileo, 2005). Avoiding terms that indicate absolutes regarding the behavior (e.g., "always") may make the story more generalizable across a variety of settings and interaction opportunities.

Once the Social Story or social narrative is written, visuals should be added to the story. Pictures should support textual information presented in the Social Story or social narrative. They should encapsulate essential elements of the story while avoiding presenting additional, non-critical information. Pictures could be photographs, icons, or drawn images. Once pictures are selected that support the story, the story can be formatted. No more than one directive sentence should be presented per page, with approximately one to three descriptive or perspective sentences per page—with accompanying picture (Crozier & Sileo, 2005).

At this point in time, the Social Story or social narrative is considered to be complete and implementation of the intervention can be commenced. Similar to video models, there is not a clear guide in terms of the frequency that a learner should read a Social Story or social narrative. Many authors recommend reviewing the Social Story or social narrative immediately before the behavior is expected to be demonstrated. For example, if the story describes skills to be used at recess, then the story should be reviewed immediately before recess. Initially, the learner should read the Social Story or social narrative with the interventionist. The interventionist should then ask comprehension questions to ensure that the learner attended to and understood the story. It may also be beneficial for the interventionist and learner to role-play the behavior after reading the Social Story or social narrative, providing the learner with an opportunity to practice and gain experience in use of the skill.

As stated above, the research is inconclusive regarding a dosage of Social Story or social narratives that is beneficial for all learners. Some learners may require daily reading of the story over an extended period of time, whereas others may acquire and demonstrate skill use rapidly. Because of this, it is critical that data be continually collected to determine whether the intervention is producing the intended effect or whether modifications to intervention procedures are warranted. Should data show a lack of response, interventionists may consider increasing the intensity of intervention procedures (e.g., reviewing the social story more often) or whether additional intervention strategies should be incorporated (e.g., provision of reinforcement for skill demonstration in the target setting).

As with any intervention, it is critical that interventionists consider how intervention effects may be maintained over time and generalized to other contexts. Should data indicate that the Social Story or social narrative is effective, the interventionist may consider systematically decreasing the frequency with which the story is read. It is recommended that decreasing frequency of supports be done carefully, avoiding a loss of intervention process by removing intervention supports too rapidly. Earlier, it was recommended that Social Stories or social narratives avoid the use of absolute terminology so as to allow for flexibility in use of the story and in demonstration of the skill. Interventionists may also plan for generalization of skills through strategies such as mediating generalization (Stokes & Baer, 1977), explicitly teaching the learner to self-monitor their use of the skill, and providing reinforcement for generalized skill use.

Practical Case Example

Jensen is an 8-year-old student in first grade. His teacher has reported that Jensen has difficulty taking turns during recess, with peers complaining that Jensen will not let them participate in activities. His teacher consulted with a school psychologist, who recommended that a Social Story intervention may be beneficial. After Jensen's caregiver consented to the intervention being implemented, Jensen's teacher and the school psychologist developed a definition of turn taking. Turn taking was described as Jensen providing opportunities for peers to participate in an activity following his turn. Through an interview and brief observation, the school psychologist generated a hypothesis regarding Jensen's behavior: that it was maintained by access to tangible objects (e.g., playground/sports equipment).

Three observations were then conducted during Jensen's regularly scheduled recess periods. These observations revealed that Jensen demonstrated zero instances of turn taking during any recess period. The school psychologist then wrote a social story, incorporating descriptive, directive, perspective, and control sentences.

At my school, kids play games at recess. Kids often use equipment like balls and jump ropes to play games at recess. When I go to recess, I can share my equipment with other kids. When someone asks to play with the equipment, they may use it for a moment and then give it to me for another turn. Taking turns can be hard, but it makes everyone feel good. Kids think it is fun to take turns because it lets everyone have a chance to play. I will remember to take turns by thinking about my book about cars. Cars stop at stop signs and take turns crossing the intersection.

The school psychologist put one to two sentences on each page of the Social Story, finding a picture to go with each group of text. For the final page, the school psychologist took a picture of Jensen's book about cars. To begin intervention, Jensen's teacher read the Social Story with him. After reading the story, his teacher asked Jensen "What can you do when someone asks to play with recess equipment?" and "How can you remember to take turns?" Jensen was able to respond accurately to these questions. Following, Jensen's teacher presented the story to him immediately prior to each recess period. After reading the social story, he would return the book to his teacher and go outside to recess. Observations continued to be conducted during recess periods to determine if the intervention was effective. Data collected indicated a gradual increase in the frequency of turn taking during recess periods, increasing to an average of six instances per recess period. Anecdotally, Jensen's teacher noted that he appeared more engaged with peers and received fewer complaints from peers regarding Jensen's turn taking behavior. Jensen continued to read the social story before each recess for 2 weeks, at which point the frequency with which the social story was presented was decreased to three times per week and then once per week. Jensen's level of turn taking was maintained at recess during this time.

Jensen's teacher would remind Jensen of the Social Story during other activities in which turn taking might be expected, such as reading with partners and art. Specifically, she would remind Jensen that he could use the same turn taking skills as he did at recess. Jensen's teacher noted increased instances of turn taking across all classroom activities, with turn taking no longer being a salient concern after approximately 1 month. During the remainder of the school year, Jensen's teacher would reference the Social Story if she observed difficulty with turn taking—with Jensen being responsive to the reminder without rereading the story.

Conclusion

Social narrative strategies are lightweight antecedent interventions that have been used for decades to promote appropriate social behavior among individuals with ASD. Although a series of systematic reviews and meta-analyses are conflicted in their appraisal of social narratives as an evidence-based strategy, there is more than enough evidence to support their continued evaluation and use in this context. Practitioners are encouraged to consider important moderating factors when crafting and implementing social narratives such as the behavior being targeted, who is reading the social narrative, and the implementation setting. Social narratives represent an appealing alternative to prompt social skill acquisition when behavioral skills training may not be available and when increased client involvement in the intervention development process is warranted.

References

Coogle, C. G., Ahmed, S., Aljaffal, M. A., Alsheef, M. Y., & Hamdi, H. A. (2018). Social narrative strategies to support children with autism spectrum disorder. *Early Childhood Education Journal, 46*, 445–450.

Crozier, S., & Sileo, N. M. (2005). Encouraging positive behavior with social stories: An intervention for children with autism spectrum disorders. *Teaching Exceptional Children, 37*, 26–31.

Gray, C. (1998). Social stories 101. *The Morning News, 10*, 2–6.

Gray, C. (2000). *The new social story book*. Future Horizons.

Gray, C. A., & Garand, J. D. (1993). Social stories: Improving responses of students with autism with accurate social information. *Focus on Autistic Behavior, 8*, 1–10.

Iwata, B. A., Dorsey, M. F., Slifer, K. J., Bauman, K. E., & Richman, G. S. (1994). Toward a functional analysis of self-injury. *Journal of Applied Behavior Analysis, 27*, 197–209.

Kokina, A., & Kern, L. (2010). Social Story™ interventions for students with autism spectrum disorders: A meta-analysis. *Journal of Autism and Developmental Disorders, 40*, 812–826.

Lindsley, O. R. (1991). From technical jargon to plain English for application. *Journal of Applied Behavior Analysis, 24*, 449–458.

Morris, B. K. (2021, September 8). *Social stories*. Synapse. Retrieved from http://www.autism-help.org/communication-social-stories-autism.htm

Qi, C. H., Barton, E. E., Collier, M., Lin, Y. L., & Montoya, C. (2018). A systematic review of effects of social stories interventions for individuals with autism spectrum disorder. *Focus on Autism and Other Developmental Disabilities, 33*, 25–34.

Reynhout, G., & Carter, M. (2007). Social Story™ efficacy with a child with autism spectrum disorder and moderate intellectual disability. *Focus on Autism and Other Developmental Disabilities, 22*, 173–181.

Rose, E. (2020). *Using the power card strategy to increase social skills: A systematic review*. Doctoral dissertation, Temple University, ProQuest Dissertation Publishing.

Stokes, T. F., & Baer, D. M. (1977). An implicit technology of generalization. *Journal of Applied Behavior Analysis, 10*, 349–367.

Swaggart, B. L., Gagnon, E., Bock, S. J., Earles, T. L., Quinn, C., Myles, B. S., & Simpson, R. L. (1995). Using social stories to teach social and behavioral skills to children with autism. *Focus on Autistic Behavior, 10*, 1–16.

Test, D. W., Richter, S., Knight, V., & Spooner, F. (2011). A comprehensive review and meta-analysis of the social stories literature. *Focus on Autism and Other Developmental Disabilities, 26*, 49–62.

Chapter 6
Peer-Mediated Teaching

Within the context of social skills teaching, peer-mediated teaching refers to a subset of strategies that rely on the involvement of one or more peers to target acquisition and performance goals. More broadly, peer-mediated interventions (PMIs) are a class of intervention that recruit peers to promote behavior change across a much broader range of outcomes. Kohler and Strain (1990) describe four subtypes of peer-mediated interventions: peer tutoring, group contingencies, peer management, and peer modeling. Peer tutoring, by definition, seeks to promote academic outcomes (e.g., reading fluency, spelling accuracy) and thus is not often used to promote social skills learning; however, there is evidence to suggest that engaging in a peer tutoring paradigm may confer some social and behavioral benefit to the tutor and tutee (e.g., Locke & Fuchs, 1995; Plumer & Stoner, 2005). Further, others have called for an expansion of its scope to address behavioral outcomes (Gumpel & Frank, 1999), blurring the lines between peer tutoring and other PMIs.

Group contingencies, the second subtype of PMIs, apply a single reinforcement contingency to a group of individuals in the hopes of modifying behavior more efficiently than many individual contingencies. Unlike peer tutoring, group contingencies often target behavioral (rather than academic) outcomes; however, the involvement of peers is less structured than the other PMI subtypes. Further, group contingencies are limited in the extent to which they promote equitable change across an entire group, often allowing one or a few individuals to satisfy the contingency for group members, depending on the type of contingency that is arranged. For this reason, they may not be ideal when the goal is to promote targeted skill acquisition or performance among a single individual or a select group. Nonetheless, group contingencies are overwhelmingly effective in promoting positive behavior change and have decades of literature to support their use across settings and populations (e.g., Little et al., 2015; Maggin et al., 2012, 2017) and they may be best used to promote broad increases in appropriate social behavior for typically developing individuals and individuals with behavioral disorders.

K. C Radley, E. H. Dart, *Social Skills Teaching for Individuals with Autism*,
Springer Series on Child and Family Studies,
https://doi.org/10.1007/978-3-030-91665-7_6

The remaining two PMI subtypes, peer modeling and peer management, have been used much more frequently than the other two (i.e., peer tutoring and group contingencies) to promote the acquisition and performance of social skills for individuals with ASD. Additionally, a third strategy, peer initiation training, involves peer interventionists but does not fit neatly into any of the four PMI subtypes. Thus, the remainder of the chapter will focus on these strategies.

Peer Modeling

Peer modeling comprises a range of procedures in which a peer is taught to exhibit specific social behaviors in the presence of learners with ASD. Video modeling (see Chap. 3) might be considered a subset of peer modeling interventions if the model depicted in the video could be reasonably construed as a peer. Otherwise, peer modeling commonly occurs live and in real time. Within peer modeling arrangements, peers are typically prompted by adult interventionists to exhibit a particular social skill and contact reinforcement for doing so appropriately. Thus, the success of a peer modeling program is dependent on individuals who can successfully exhibit the skill to be taught when prompted to do so. Like video modeling, peer modeling relies on social learning theory (Bandura & McClelland, 1977) to drive responding. Further, because peer modeling involves at least one of the components of behavioral skills training (BST; see Chap. 4), it is effective as an acquisition strategy. That is, peer models provide a demonstration of the skill to be taught and often are provided with feedback by the adult interventionist, allowing the learner to benefit observationally from at least two of the four BST components.

One of the earliest demonstrations of peer modeling for social behavior was reported by Charlop and Walsh (1986), who used it to promote spontaneous displays of verbal affection among young boys with ASD. Notably, the peer models in this study were also children with ASD who had previously acquired the target skill. Charlop and Walsh (1986) prompted learners to attend to a peer model, who was then prompted to exhibit a verbal display of affection and reinforced with a snack and social reinforcement for doing so. Next, the learner was prompted to exhibit the behavior that they just observed being exhibited by the model. Overall, they found that the learners benefitted from the peer modeling paradigm by exhibiting appropriate verbal affection which generalized across settings.

More recently, Jones and Schwartz (2004) arranged small groups of preschool aged children, only one of whom had a diagnosis of ASD, and had an adult interventionist ask "Wh-" questions (e.g., "What is this person doing?") to the typically developing group members. Correct responses by the typically developing group members contacted social reinforcement from the adult interventionist to promote observational learning before the child with ASD was posed similar questions. They found that this peer modeling procedure increased the number of correct responses to questions exhibited by the children with ASD, even after the model was no longer present, suggesting the results may have maintained over time. Interestingly, Jones and Schwartz (2004) also found that learners exhibited similar levels of accuracy across three different model types (i.e., sibling, non-sibling peer, adult), suggesting all three may be effective interventionists in this capacity when available.

Peer Management

Peer management describes any intervention strategy in which a peer is responsible for managing a contingency that is designed to modify the behavior of a learner. Additionally, peer management interventions focus exclusively on behavioral outcomes (rather than academic), distinguishing them from peer tutoring. Like the other peer-mediated strategies, peer management has been used to target a much broader scope of outcome and populations than social skills for individuals with ASD. For example, Dart et al. (2014) synthesized the school-based peer management literature and found that students with behavioral disorders and typically developing students were frequent targets of these strategies to prompt appropriate classroom behavior, communication, and social skills. Unlike peer modeling, peer management strategies place an individual within a more active and direct interventionist role. These roles often include responsibilities such as prompting, data collection, contingency management, providing feedback, and reinforcer delivery.

As an illustrative example, consider the study conducted by Ganz et al. (2012), who trained a typically developing middle school student to use a most-to-least prompting procedure to promote appropriate communicative responses made by a learner with ASD. During the intervention, the peer was responsible for providing verbal and gestural prompts to the learner to refer to a social script. The peer interventionist was also instructed to arrange situations for social interaction to take place during an arts and craft activity. This relatively simple intervention was effective, promoting increases in three different communicative behaviors (i.e., asking questions, praise, and requesting help). Although generalization of these increases to an untrained peer was not readily observed, the learner's behavior under the effects of the intervention was comparable to their typically developing peers, lending evidence to the social validity of the procedures.

In another example, Morrison et al. (2001) examined a short phase of peer monitoring, whereby typically developing elementary and middle school aged students were asked to record the frequency with which learners with ASD in their classrooms exhibited specific social behaviors (i.e., requesting, commenting, sharing). Additionally, the peers were responsible for delivering a small edible or tangible reinforcing stimulus after each occurrence of appropriate social behavior exhibited by the learners. Although not directly related to the primary aims and outcomes of the intervention, the peers were also eligible to receive reinforcement for correctly implementing the peer monitoring procedures. The authors found that the peer monitoring procedure was as least as effective than a self-monitoring procedure in all cases and far superior to a no treatment baseline. Although they noted that self-monitoring might be preferable due to its ability to promote independence, the peer monitoring strategy investigated here may promote greater generalization of the learned skills across other peers.

The meta-analysis by Dart et al. (2014) also identified a number of other factors to consider when developing peer management interventions. First, they found that gender-matched peers and learners produced slightly greater intervention effects than pairs that were not matched by gender. Second, they found that interventionist-learner pairs that shared a classroom produced slightly greater intervention effects than those that did not. Finally, they noted that longer peer training requirements (i.e., greater than 60 min) produced substantially greater treatment effects than interventions requiring shorter training (i.e., less than or equal to 60 min). Together, these findings suggest that gender-matched peers sharing an environment (e.g., a classroom) where the peer interventionist receives high duration training on the peer management procedures is likely to produce the most effective outcomes.

Peer Initiation Training

The final peer-mediated strategy to promote social skills in individuals with ASD is peer initiation training. Within this strategy, peer interventionists are taught only to initiate social interaction with a learner with ASD. Peer initiation training is distinct from peer modeling, which involves demonstration but not necessarily interaction, and peer management, which involves interventionist interaction but in a greater capacity than simply initiating social contact. Peer initiation training promotes performance of social behaviors by providing learners with many more opportunities to respond to social situations than they would typically otherwise receive. Further, peer initiation training can be coupled with other strategies such as performance feedback and behavioral skills training to address possible acquisition deficits. Due to its flexibility, peer initiating training is a valuable strategy and commonly used in a wide variety of settings.

An early example by Odom and Strain (1986) compared a peer initiation strategy to a teacher antecedent strategy to promote social interaction among preschool children with ASD. Four typically developing preschool children were taught to approach and initiate social interactions with the target students in a way that would encourage prolonged interaction. The intervention was implemented during a 15-min free play time within the preschool classroom. The authors found that the peer initiation training was superior to the teacher antecedent condition in promoting appropriate social responses by the target students; however, they found that the teacher antecedent strategy was more effective in promoting learners' social initiations.

Identifying Peers

Although it may vary across contexts, the definition of a peer within the context of PMIs can be broad but usually refers to an individual near or at the same age of the learner and with similar social standing. For example, PMI work in schools may identify a peer as a student within the same classroom (e.g., Grauvogel-MacAleese & Wallace, 2010) or school building (e.g., Dart et al., 2015) as the learner. PMIs in clinical settings may recruit siblings (e.g., Flood et al., 2002) or individuals from the community (e.g., Corbett et al., 2014) as intervention agents. For practical purposes, the peers should be regularly available to engage in the intervention work and capable of managing the responsibility of implementation, whatever that may look like. As mentioned previously, for peer modeling interventions, the peers should be able to demonstrate the skills being taught. For peer management interventions, the peers should be able to manage a reinforcement contingency and be prepared to interact directly with the learner in an appropriate manner.

Identifying peers to serve in a management, modeling, or initiation capacity involves consideration of several important factors. First, the method of identification may vary but is often accomplished through parent or teacher referral (e.g., Morrison et al., 2001). Keep in mind that referrals may be subject to biases so it may be beneficial to provide potential referrers with objective standards or criteria by which they consider individuals for a peer interventionist role. Previous researchers have used characteristic checklists (e.g., Dart et al., 2015) to ensure that peer interventionists are deemed to possess one or more subjective qualities that are considered desirable (e.g., kind, compassionate, responsible). Odom (2019) recommended that peer interventionists share some similarities with the learners they are engaging and that the ratio of peer interventionist to learner is greater than 1:1 to avoid fatigue or peer burnout. Finally, if you are seeking the participation of minor children as peer interventionists, make sure that the appropriate consent and assent procedures are in place before beginning work in this way.

Strain and Kohler (1998) provide several additional thoughts regarding the use of peer-mediated interventions for promoting social behavior in individuals with ASD. First, they note that the research supporting these strategies provides sufficient evidence that highly structured adult-driven interventions may not be necessary to accomplish these treatment goals. Second, they advocate for developmental integration, meaning learners with ASD are provided with instruction and opportunities to interact with peers in a fully integrated setting to promote skill acquisition, generalization, and enhance social development. Third, they emphasize the importance of treatment fidelity, or the degree to which the intervention is implemented as intended. Treatment fidelity may be particularly important to monitor when engaging in peer-mediated work as the primary interventionists may not be a credentialed professional with many years of experience. Finally, they state that the peer-mediated intervention process confers benefits upon the peer interventionist, similar to the effects observed within the peer tutoring process. Next, we will provide a brief review of the empirical evidence supporting peer-mediated strategies to promote social skill acquisition and maintenance for individuals with ASD.

Empirical Basis of Peer-Mediated Intervention

Peer-mediated interventions represent one of the more frequently researched social skills teaching strategies. In a review of single-case research published between 1998 and 2018 conducted by Radley et al. (2020), peer-mediated interventions represented the fourth most frequently researched social skills teaching intervention strategy. Radley et al. reported that research in peer-mediated interventions generally adhered to design standards, included participants of a wide range of ages, and most typically evaluated intervention effects on social engagement of participants.

General Effectiveness of Peer-Mediated Interventions

Several researchers have conducted meta-analyses or systematic reviews of peer-mediated social skills teaching interventions, providing summaries of the effects of participation in such interventions. Watkins et al. (2015) conducted a systematic review, identifying 14 studies including 44 participants with ASD and over 130 typically developing peers. The review documented interventions occurring in a variety of locations (e.g., playground, classroom), with most studies focusing on teaching peer initiation strategies to typically developing peers (i.e., 10 of 14 studies). Although no quantitative estimate of effect was provided as part of the review, Watkins et al. report that 10 of the studies documented positive outcomes for all participants and variables assessed, with the remaining four studies showing generally positive, albeit mixed, results. Further, despite not conducting analyses considering level of functioning as a moderator of intervention effect, Watkins et al. reported that most studies identified included individuals with ASD who were reported to have an IQ above 55—suggesting the need for additional evaluation of the utility of peer-mediated social skills teaching interventions with individuals with lower functioning levels.

Although not specific to social skills teaching, Chan et al. (2009) provided an additional systematic review of peer-mediated intervention for individuals with ASD. Across 42 studies identified, social skills outcomes were the most frequently assessed—representing 88% of studies evaluating peer-mediated intervention. In providing a summary of intervention findings, Chan et al. indicate that over 90% of studies reported positive results, with no studies indicating negative findings. Of particular note are studies identified (e.g., Carter et al., 2005) which identified positive outcomes for both participants with ASD and peer interventionists. In further emphasizing the potential utility of peer-mediated interventions, studies reporting social validity generally documented acceptability of procedures and effectiveness for both target students and peers.

Several meta-analyses have explicitly evaluated the effects of peer-mediated intervention for individuals with ASD, whereas others have included peer-mediated interventions as part of a broader evaluation of the effect of social skills teaching for individuals with ASD. Bene et al. (2014) conducted a meta-analysis of single-case design research of peer-mediated interventions targeting academic and social skills of individuals with ASD, identifying 14 studies. Whereas some of the studies assessed only academic outcomes, several studies assessed social outcomes in participants. Using nonoverlap of all pairs (Parker & Vannest, 2009) as a measure of effect, a score of 0.83 was reported for social and behavioral outcomes—interpreted as a strong effect. No differences in effect were found across ages of participants, with peer-mediated interventions being generally effective for all participants.

Zhang and Wheeler (2011) also conducted a meta-analysis of peer-mediated interventions, focusing specifically on social outcomes of interventions. A total of 20 studies, published between 1978 and 2006, were identified for inclusion in the meta-analysis. Results of the meta-analysis found peer-mediated interventions to result in large interventions for frequency and duration of social engagement. Analyses indicated that peer-mediated interventions were highly effective across participant age, gender, or diagnosis, as well as across peer interventionist age or gender. Siblings were found to be among the most effective peer interventionists, with home-based intervention being more effective than interventions conducted in other settings. Although peer-mediated interventions were generally found to be effective, peer modeling, in which a peer demonstrated the target social skill, was found to be substantially more effective than other types of peer-mediated interventions.

In a meta-analysis of peer-mediated and video modeling social skills interventions for individuals with ASD, Wang et al. (2011) identified nine studies that utilized peer-mediated intervention to deliver social skills teaching. Results of the meta-analysis revealed that peer-mediated intervention and video modeling interventions produced similar effects (i.e., both interventions were equally effective). Effects reported were interpreted as large (Cohen, 1988). Similar to Bene et al. (2014) no clear effects of age were identified; however, it should be noted that studies represented a restricted age range (i.e., no studies with participants over age 10 were identified for inclusion in the meta-analysis). Overall, Wang et al. (2011) suggest that the results indicate that peer-mediated intervention should be considered an evidence-based intervention for social skills teaching.

Watkins et al. (2017) conducted a meta-analyses of single-case research for school-based interventions for adolescents with ASD. A total of 27 studies were identified as meeting inclusion criteria, 10 of which evaluated peer-mediated social skills teaching interventions. Although the largest effect sizes were observed for teacher-implemented interventions, peers were still found to result in large intervention effects—with the quantitative estimate of peer-mediated intervention being greater than that for researcher-implemented interventions. Intervention effect was not found to vary substantially with level of participant functioning, suggesting the utility of peer-mediated social skills teaching strategies across participants. These results were replicated in a follow-up meta-analysis (Watkins et al., 2019), with peer-mediated interventions again being found to be effective—with study authors concluding that peer-mediated interventions should be considered recommended social skills teaching interventions.

Finally, the National Standards Project (2015) has provided a summary of the evidence-base for peer-mediated interventions for children with ASD. In synthesizing 46 studies including children between the ages of 3 and 14, it was concluded that peer-mediated interventions represented an established intervention for children with ASD.

Specific Outcomes

Peer-mediated interventions have been used to target a wide range of social skills. For example, Trembath et al. (2009) evaluated peer-mediated intervention as a strategy for improving communicative behaviors using an augmentative and alternative communication device—with communication increasing following implementation of the peer-mediated intervention. In another study, peer-mediated intervention was used to teach joint attention skills (Ferraioli & Harris, 2011). Intervention focused on an eight-step joint attention procedure, with peer-mediated intervention implemented by a sibling being effective in increasing accuracy of skill demonstration. Further, intervention was found to result in increases in spontaneous target imitation across participants—despite social imitation not being a primary focus of the intervention.

Although peer-mediated interventions are applicable to a wide range of non-social (e.g., academic tasks) and social skill outcomes, the majority of research has more narrowly focused on social engagement as the primary outcome of intervention. In Radley et al.'s (2020) review, of the 28 peer-mediated social skills teaching interventions identified, 21 (75%) of studies assessed social engagement as a primary outcome. This finding is consistent with other research identifying social engagement or social interaction as a primary outcome for peer-mediated intervention (e.g., Watkins et al., 2015), and is likely the result of the nature of peer-mediated intervention which inherently programs for interaction between peers and individuals with ASD. Overall, research has supported the utility of peer-mediated interventions in promoting social engagement, which may be considered a particularly socially valid outcome for individuals with ASD given that they have been found to initiate interactions less frequently than peers (e.g., Bauminger et al., 2003) and may miss bids for interactions from others (e.g., Meindl & Cannella-Malone, 2011).

Considering initiations as a core element of social engagement, a number of studies have specifically evaluated the effect of peer-mediated social skills teaching on social interactions of individuals with ASD. In one example, Simpson and Bui (2016) implemented an intervention in which peers provided a reading intervention (i.e., "Reading Buddies") to students with ASD. Peers were instructed to perform three general steps to implement the intervention: staying near their buddy, reading with their buddy, and talking with their buddy. Following implementation of the intervention, both participants with ASD and peer interventionists were found to demonstrate a greater number of social initiations. Additional data were collected that demonstrated social validity of intervention procedures, with peers indicating that they enjoyed participating in the intervention and participants indicated that they appreciated the friendship they had with their peer.

In another study, Hu et al. (2018) implemented a peer-mediated play intervention including 3 children with ASD and 13 peers. Peers were taught a variety of skills to facilitate interactions with participants with ASD, including naming LEGO pieces and building skills, response and initiation skills, and modeling building actions and prompting peers. During each intervention session, one participant with ASD and two peers engaged in building a LEGO model, with each individual performing a different role in accomplishing the task. Following implementation of the intervention, the number of social interactions of participants with ASD was found to increase across all participants, with teacher report indicating that participants with ASD demonstrated more interest in peers and interacted with them with greater frequency.

Social responses to peers' bids for attention also appear to be impacted by peer-mediated social skills teaching interventions. Dueñas et al. (2021) implemented a multicomponent peer-mediated intervention, consisting of both peer self-management and video modeling, with three young children with ASD and three typically developing peers. The peer self-management portion of the intervention consisted of having typically developing peers record the extent to which they appropriately responded to initiations from peers with ASD using a video recorded during baseline. More specifically, peers recorded the frequency of looking in the direction of the participant with ASD when socially initiated, staying nearby, listening, and responding within 5-s of the initiation. Once implemented, rapid increases in the number of social responses of participants with ASD were observed. Data on social initiations were also collected; however, these demonstrated more limited improvements compared to changes in social responses. Overall, the frequency of social communication exchanges was observed to increase across all participants with ASD.

In a study conducted by Sutton et al. (2021), social interaction centers were embedded within four elementary school classrooms. Five individuals with ASD were included within the classrooms. During the intervention, the participants with ASD and their classroom peers were provided with structured opportunities to engage in social communication about books. For all participants with ASD, implementation of the intervention resulted in increases in the number of social responses per minute, as well as increases in on-topic initiations and decreases in off-topic initiations. Further, these effects were maintained over time—providing additional evidence regarding the utility of peer-mediated intervention as a means of promoting social responses of participants.

Combining both social initiations and responses, researchers have demonstrated that peer-mediated interventions can be effective in increasing the overall social engagement of individuals with ASD. For example, Brain and Mirenda (2019) provided nine typically developing peers with 40–50 min of coaching, during which they were encouraged to interact with their peers with ASD during lunch breaks using specific interaction strategies. Peers were also provided with ongoing feedback regarding use of skills during lunch break periods. Following implementation of the intervention, the duration of time in which three individuals with ASD spent engaged with peers increased substantially—with all participants showing zero levels of engagement during baseline to participants approaching 100% engagement during intervention. Further, increases in indicators of mutual enjoyment (e.g., laughing, smiling) were observed to be high during intervention and follow-up phases. Peers also reported satisfaction with intervention procedures, with participants reporting that they considered their classmate to be a friend and that they enjoyed participation in the intervention.

Resources and Practical Guide

There are a number of resources available to practitioners wishing to implement peer-mediated interventions with their clients. First, Collins and Hawkins (2020) published an edited book that serves as a practical guide to implementing peer-mediated interventions in a school setting. Although it is meant for school-based practitioners and does not exclusively focus on individuals with ASD, the text nonetheless contains a wealth of useful information related to every aspect of peer-mediated interventions with chapters dedicated to peer management, peer modeling, and peer-mediated social skills training. Battaglia and Radley (2014) also provide a more succinct practical guide to peer-mediated interventions focusing specifically on those designed to promote social skill acquisition and performance in individuals with ASD. They outline four discrete steps of the peer-mediated intervention process as well as provide two case examples of the steps in action.

The first step recommended by Battaglia and Radley (2014) is to identify the peers who will be a part of the intervention process. In addition to the information we have already reviewed about identifying peers earlier in this chapter, they note that peers should have a positive or neutral history with the learners with whom they will interact. Further, they suggest that peers be willing to participate in the intervention procedures. With this recommendation in mind, we encourage practitioners not to undervalue the child assent process. In other words, if a minor peer states that they are not interested or willing to participate in the intervention process, even if you have received parental consent for them to participate, you should not move forward with that individual as a peer interventionist.

Second, Battaglia and Radley (2014) recommend identifying the skill to be targeted and collect baseline data on that skill. We touched on this process in Chap. 2 when we discussed assessment of social skills and the information provided by the authors is largely consistent. They recommend some combination of rating scale, interview, and direct observation data to identify skill or performance deficits followed by a brief monitoring period with no intervention in place to identify present levels of functioning and confirm that a deficit is in fact present. Although this step is no different for peer-mediated interventions than it is for any other class of interventions, it is no less important. Further, it may be useful to conduct assessment of the peer interventionists' social behavior during this time to confirm that they have the prerequisite skills to engage in the intervention work.

Third, practitioners are guided to choose and implement one of the many peer-mediated intervention strategies available. Battaglia and Radley (2014) recommend peer initiation training to address performance deficits and peer modeling or peer management to address acquisition deficits. Further, some consideration of the resources available to implement one or more strategies is necessary to determine which will be possible or feasible. Keep in mind that it will be necessary to allocate time to training the peer interventionist prior to implementation. Additionally, identify as many potential peer interventionists as possible to increase the likelihood that one or more make it through the consent, assent, and training process and to account for unanticipated absences or other forms of attrition.

Finally, Battaglia and Radley (2014) recommend monitoring the progress of the intervention strategy once it is being implemented to determine whether it is effective. Again, although this information was discussed in Chap. 2, they provide some additional considerations unique to peer-mediated interventions. For example, if during the monitoring process the intervention is deemed ineffective, consider whether it is due to the specific peer interventionist(s) who are responsible for implementation. Alternatively, it may be that the peer interventionists' implementation fidelity is poor and that they need to be retrained. This may be particularly difficult to identify if you are relying on peer self-report of implementation and not engaging in direct observation. Consider using multiple methods of treatment fidelity assessment to generate a robust estimate of implementation behavior.

Practical Case Example

Calvin is a 5-year-old male who receives special education services under the category of Autism. Calvin's teacher has reported that he often observes other peers during recess periods but rarely plays or engages with others in the class during those times. In collaboration with the special education team and Calvin's guardian, it was determined that support should be provided during recess that would facilitate Calvin's engagement with peers. Stakeholders believed that recess would provide ample opportunities for Calvin to practice communication skills in unstructured settings, supporting other Individualized Education Plan goals.

To identify supports that might be beneficial, observations were conducted during recess periods. These observations revealed that Calvin would typically stand near peer groups and observe play activities. However, Calvin was only observed to initiate an interaction and join a group on one occasion. In discussing the results of observations with the special education team, Calvin's teacher indicated that Calvin typically will engage in observation of preferred peers. In collaborating, a peer-mediated intervention incorporating preferred peers was suggested as a possible support for recess periods. It was decided a recess buddy group, including Calvin and some preferred peers, would be implemented.

The school psychologist sent consent forms home to Calvin and teacher-identified peers to be part of a recess buddy group. Consent forms described the purpose of the group as a skills-based group in which kids would learn friendship and problem-solving skills. Of the seven consent forms sent home to peers, four were returned with consent to participate. Calvin's guardian also returned a consent to participate in the group. Next, the school psychologist identified skills that would be covered in the group. Initially, the school psychologist identified three skills to be taught: joining a group, inviting others to play, and deciding on an activity collaboratively. Task analyses were developed for the three skills, and a weekly recess period was identified for implementation of the intervention.

During each peer buddy group, Calvin and his peers would meet with the school psychologist on the playground during recess. The school psychologist would briefly describe the target skill and the steps to skill completion. Next, participants in the group would practice the skill in the context of recess activities. For example, group members practiced joining in an activity in the context of a game of tag. Each lesson took the entirety of one recess period, or approximately 10 min. During other recesses, the school psychologist would observe skill use of Calvin and his peers. When Calvin was observed to regularly demonstrate the target skill during non-teaching recess periods, the next skill was introduced. This process continued until all three skills had been taught and Calvin was observed to demonstrate all skills with regularity during unstructured recess periods. In discussing the results of the intervention with Calvin's teacher, his teacher reported that Calvin was observed to be substantially more engaged with peers during recess. Calvin also reported to his guardian that he had made several new friends at school. Together, recess observation data and anecdotal reports from stakeholders were used to determine that the intervention had been beneficial in supporting Calvin during recess periods.

Conclusion

To summarize, peer-mediated strategies actually comprise a range of intervention techniques that have been used for decades to promote the acquisition and performance of both specific social skills and broader social functioning in individuals with ASD. Although these strategies are associated with some unique considerations related to the use of peers as the primary intervention agent, the flexibility, efficiency, and generalization they afford make them valuable options in this context. Practitioners operating within an environment with greater access to peers (e.g., school or community setting) are encouraged to consider peer-mediated interventions for their clients due to the benefits afforded to the learners and peer interventionists.

References

Bandura, A., & McClelland, D. C. (1977). *Social learning theory*. Prentice Hall.

Battaglia, A. A., & Radley, K. C. (2014). Peer-mediated social skills training for children with autism spectrum disorder. *Beyond Behavior, 23*, 4–13.

Bauminger, N., Shulman, C., & Agam, G. (2003). Peer interaction and loneliness in high-functioning children with autism. *Journal of Autism and Developmental Disorders, 33*, 489–507.

Bene, K., Banda, D. R., & Brown, D. (2014). A meta-analysis of peer-mediated instructional arrangements and autism. *Review Journal of Autism and Developmental Disorders, 1*, 135–142.

Brain, T., & Mirenda, P. (2019). Effectiveness of a low-intensity peer-mediated intervention for middle school students with autism spectrum disorder. *Research in Autism Spectrum Disorders, 62*, 26–38.

Carter, E. W., Cushing, L. S., Clark, N. M., & Kennedy, C. H. (2005). Effects of peer support interventions on students' access to the general curriculum and social interactions. *Research and Practice for Persons with Severe Disabilities, 30*, 15–25.

Chan, J. M., Lang, R., Rispoli, M., O'Reilly, M., Sigafoos, J., & Cole, H. (2009). Use of peer-mediated interventions in the treatment of autism spectrum disorders: A systematic review. *Research in Autism Spectrum Disorders, 3*, 876–889.

Charlop, M. H., & Walsh, M. E. (1986). Increasing autistic children's spontaneous verbalizations of affection: An assessment of time delay and peer modeling procedures. *Journal of Applied Behavior Analysis, 19*, 307–314.

Cohen, J. (1988). *Statistical power analysis for the behavioral sciences* (2nd ed.). Erlbaum.

Collins, T. A., & Hawkins, R. O. (Eds.). (2020). *Peers as change agents: A guide to implementing peer-mediated interventions in schools*. Oxford University Press.

Corbett, B. A., Swain, D. M., Coke, C., Simon, D., Newsom, C., Houchins-Juarez, N., et al. (2014). Improvement in social deficits in autism spectrum disorders using a theatre-based, peer-mediated intervention. *Autism Research, 7*, 4–16.

Dart, E. H., Collins, T. A., Klingbeil, D. A., & McKinley, L. E. (2014). Peer management interventions: A meta-analytic review of single-case research. *School Psychology Review, 43*, 367–384.

Dart, E. H., Furlow, C. M., Collins, T. A., Brewer, E., Gresham, F. M., & Chenier, K. H. (2015). Peer-mediated check-in/check-out for students at-risk for internalizing disorders. *School Psychology Quarterly, 30*, 229.

Dueñas, A. D., Plavnick, J. B., & Goldstein, H. (2021). Effects of a multicomponent peer mediated intervention on social communication of preschoolers with autism spectrum disorder. *Exceptional Children, 87*, 236–257.

Ferraioli, S. J., & Harris, S. L. (2011). Teaching joint attention to children with autism through a sibling-mediated behavioral intervention. *Behavioral Interventions, 26*, 261–281.

Flood, W. A., Wilder, D. A., Flood, A. L., & Masuda, A. (2002). Peer-mediated reinforcement plus prompting as treatment for off-task behavior in children with attention deficit hyperactivity disorder. *Journal of Applied Behavior Analysis, 35*, 199–204.

Ganz, J. B., Heath, A. K., Lund, E. M., Camargo, S. P., Rispoli, M. J., Boles, M., & Plaisance, L. (2012). Effects of peer-mediated implementation of visual scripts in middle school. *Behavior Modification, 36*, 378–398.

Grauvogel-MacAleese, A. N., & Wallace, M. D. (2010). Use of peer-mediated intervention in children with attention deficit hyperactivity disorder. *Journal of Applied Behavior Analysis, 43*, 547–551.

Gumpel, T. P., & Frank, R. (1999). An expansion of the peer-tutoring paradigm: Cross-age peer tutoring of social skills among socially rejected boys. *Journal of Applied Behavior Analysis, 32*, 115–118.

Hu, X., Zheng, Q., & Lee, G. T. (2018). Using peer-mediated LEGO® play intervention to improve social interactions for Chinese children with autism in an inclusive setting. *Journal of Autism and Developmental Disorders, 48*, 2444–2457.

Jones, C. D., & Schwartz, I. S. (2004). Siblings, peers, and adults: Differential effects of models for children with autism. *Topics in Early Childhood Special Education, 24*, 187–198.
Kohler, F. W., & Strain, P. S. (1990). Peer-assisted interventions: Early promises, notable achievements, and future aspirations. *Clinical Psychology Review, 22*, 441–454.
Little, S. G., Akin-Little, A., & O'Neill, K. (2015). Group contingency interventions with children—1980-2010: A meta-analysis. *Behavior Modification, 39*, 322–341.
Locke, W. R., & Fuchs, L. S. (1995). Effects of peer-mediated reading instruction on the on-task behavior and social interaction of children with behavior disorders. *Journal of Emotional and Behavioral Disorders, 3*, 92–99.
Maggin, D. M., Johnson, A. H., Chafouleas, S. M., Ruberto, L. M., & Berggren, M. (2012). A systematic evidence review of school-based group contingency interventions for students with challenging behavior. *Journal of School Psychology, 50*, 625–654.
Maggin, D. M., Pustejovsky, J. E., & Johnson, A. H. (2017). A meta-analysis of school-based group contingency interventions for students with challenging behavior: An update. *Remedial and Special Education, 38*, 353–370.
Meindl, J. N., & Cannella-Malone, H. I. (2011). Initiating and responding to joint attention bids in children with autism: A review of the literature. *Research in Developmental Disabilities, 32*, 1441–1454.
Morrison, L., Kamps, D., Garcia, J., & Parker, D. (2001). Peer mediation and monitoring strategies to improve initiations and social skills for students with autism. *Journal of Positive Behavior Interventions, 3*, 237–250.
National Autism Center. (2015). *Findings and conclusions: National standards project, Phase 2*. Retrieved from http://www.nationalautismcenter.org/
Odom, S. L. (2019). Peer-based interventions for children and youth with autism spectrum disorder: History and effects. *School Psychology Review, 48*, 170–176.
Odom, S. L., & Strain, P. S. (1986). A comparison of peer-initiation and teacher-antecedent interventions for promoting reciprocal social interaction of autistic preschoolers. *Journal of Applied Behavior Analysis, 19*, 59–71.
Parker, R. I., & Vannest, K. (2009). An improved effect size for single-case research: Nonoverlap of all pairs. *Behavior Therapy, 40*, 357–367.
Plumer, P. J., & Stoner, G. (2005). The relative effects of classwide peer tutoring and peer coaching on the positive social behaviors of children with ADHD. *Journal of Attention Disorders, 9*, 290–300.
Radley, K. C., Dart, E. H., Fischer, A. J., & Collins, T. A. (2020). Publication trends for single-case methodology in school psychology: A systematic review. *Psychology in the Schools, 57*, 683–698.
Simpson, L. A., & Bui, Y. (2016). Effects of a peer-mediated intervention on social interactions of students with low-functioning autism and perceptions of typical peers. *Education and Training in Autism and Developmental Disabilities*, 162–178.
Strain, P. S., & Kohler, F. (1998). Peer-mediated social intervention for young children with autism. In *Seminars in speech and language* (Vol. 19, No. 04, pp. 391–405). © 1998 by Thieme Medical Publishers, Inc.
Sutton, B. M., Westerveld, M. F., & Webster, A. A. (2021). Classroom teachers' implementation of the social stations intervention to improve the verbal initiations and responses of students with autism. *Journal of Autism and Developmental Disorders*, 1–15.
Trembath, D., Balandin, S., Togher, L., & Stancliffe, R. J. (2009). Peer-mediated teaching and augmentative and alternative communication for preschool-aged children with autism. *Journal of Intellectual and Developmental Disability, 34*, 173–186.
Wang, S. Y., Cui, Y., & Parrila, R. (2011). Examining the effectiveness of peer-mediated and video-modeling social skills interventions for children with autism spectrum disorders: A meta-analysis in single-case research using HLM. *Research in Autism Spectrum Disorders, 5*, 562–569.

Watkins, L., Ledbetter-Cho, K., O'Reilly, M., Barnard-Brak, L., & Garcia-Grau, P. (2019). Interventions for students with autism in inclusive settings: A best-evidence synthesis and meta-analysis. *Psychological Bulletin, 145*, 490–507.
Watkins, L., O'Reilly, M., Kuhn, M., Gevarter, C., Lancioni, G. E., Sigafoos, J., & Lang, R. (2015). A review of peer-mediated social interaction interventions for students with autism in inclusive settings. *Journal of Autism and Developmental Disorders, 45*, 1070–1083.
Watkins, L., O'Reilly, M., Ledbetter-Cho, K., Lang, R., Sigafoos, J., Kuhn, M., et al. (2017). A meta-analysis of school-based social interaction interventions for adolescents with autism spectrum disorder. *Review Journal of Autism and Developmental Disorders, 4*, 277–293.
Zhang, J., & Wheeler, J. J. (2011). A meta-analysis of peer-mediated interventions for young children with autism spectrum disorders. *Education and Training in Autism and Developmental Disabilities, 46*, 62–77.

Chapter 7
Antecedent Interventions

Behaviors are often conceptualized using the three-term contingency, or ABCs of behavior: antecedent-behavior-consequence (Moxley, 1996). Using this conceptualization, social skills teaching strategies may generally be classified as aiming to affect a relevant dimension of a behavior *prior* to the behavior occurring (i.e., antecedent intervention), or to affect future occurrences of a behavior through delivery of a consequence following demonstration of a behavior—typically through delivery of positive reinforcement (e.g., Cooper et al., 2020). Using this definition, a majority of social skills teaching strategies could likely be considered antecedent strategies. Indeed, previous meta-analyses and reviews have used such a definition in classifying social skills teaching strategies (e.g., Ledford et al., 2018).

Other research has provided a more narrow definition of antecedent strategies. For example, Radley and Dart (2016) describe antecedent interventions as a class of intervention in which environmental modifications are made that may impact the occurrence of a target behavior. Examples of strategies that may meet this definition include setting up an environment in a particular way to facilitate social skill use or to train interactional strategies to those that may engage with individuals with ASD as a means of improving social skill outcomes.

For the purposes of this chapter, antecedent interventions will be defined as strategies that are implemented prior to expected use of a social skill but *do not* involve any direct training in use of a target skill. Thus, for this chapter, strategies such as video models and social stories, which have been described as antecedent strategies (e.g., Ledford et al., 2018), are not included and are described elsewhere in this text. Using this definition, prompting and cueing interventions, visual or activity schedules, and environmental modifications (e.g., space, activities) were considered antecedent strategies and are described below.

K. C Radley, E. H. Dart, *Social Skills Teaching for Individuals with Autism*,
Springer Series on Child and Family Studies,
https://doi.org/10.1007/978-3-030-91665-7_7

Prompting and Cueing

Prompting and cueing interventions describe strategies in which an individual is provided with hints or reminders to demonstrate a skill. Within the empirical literature, the terms prompts and cues are often used interchangeably—resulting in some ambiguity in terminology. Although related to each other, prompts and cues may be differentiated by their topography. Prompts may be defined as supports that are provided to increase the success of an individual in performing some skill (e.g., Mayer et al., 2012). The prompts within a prompting intervention do not necessarily approximate the target behavior, but only serve to scaffold use of a social skill. Whereas prompts represent an artificial antecedent that is intended to promote use of a skill, cues are stimuli within the natural social environment that remind a learner to use a skill. Cues, unlike prompts, are directly related to use of the skill. In relation to prompts, cues may be considered to be the end product of a faded prompting intervention. That is, the use of a skill is no longer supported artificially, but is maintained by stimuli within the natural environment. As such, cueing interventions will not be discussed separately from prompting, but the transition from artificial prompts to natural cues for skill use should be a consideration of any social skills prompting intervention.

Prompting interventions can generally be classified by their topography, or the form in which prompts are provided. Broadly, prompting interventions may be classified as using one or more of the following types of prompts: gestural, written or verbal, model, or physical prompts. Prompts may be classified based on how intrusive they are or how much support is provided, with gestural prompts representing the lowest intensity prompt and physical prompts representing the most invasive form of prompting.

Gestural prompts are a type of prompt in which an interventionist indicates that a skill should be used through pointing or gesturing. Gestural prompts are noninvasive and should be considered a low-level type of prompt. With respect to social skills, gestural prompts could be used to signal that a learner could join in a group or invite a peer to play (e.g., pointing at a game, motioning toward a peer).

Written or verbal prompts involve the use of language to support use of a social skill. Written or verbal prompts are relatively more invasive than gestural prompts, requiring more direct interaction between the interventionist and the learner with ASD. Written or verbal prompts could also be either specific or general—providing explicit suggestions for what a learner should do (e.g., "say the peers name to get their attention") or a more general prompt to engage in a behavior (e.g., "what could you do to get their attention"). As an example of a verbal prompt, an interventionist could tell a learner to try joining a group of peers or to remember to ask a peer for help. Written prompts could entail a learner referencing a list of conversation starters for joining in a peer group or an interventionist using cue cards to suggest ideas for conversation or activities with peers.

Model prompts describe the process of an interventionist showing a learner what they should do. Relative to written or verbal prompts, model prompts are relatively more intrusive, as it requires more assistance or instruction to be provided by the interventionist. With respect to social skills, a model prompt may take the form of an interventionist showing a learner how to request help from a teacher when the learner fails to do so independently, or modeling an appropriate way to join in a group after a learner demonstrates unsuccessful joining in.

Physical prompts describe guiding a learner through completion of a task using physical guidance. Physical prompts represent the most invasive form of prompting, requiring direct physical contact between the interventionist and the learner. Physical prompts are infrequently used in the context of social skills, with these types of prompts being more regularly observed in prompting acquisition of other types of behaviors (e.g., Waters et al., 2009). Applied to social skills, an example of a physical prompt may be providing hand-over-hand guidance to the learner in raising their hand when they need help from a teacher.

Prompting interventions frequently utilize a least-to-most prompting procedure. In this, individuals are initially provided with the lowest level of prompting to support skill use (e.g., gestural), with more intensive or invasive prompts being provided only when a learner fails to respond to a lower intensity prompt. To illustrate, a social skills teaching intervention may aim to promote labeling and responding to emotions of others. After teaching general steps to the target skill, the interventionist may observe the learner use the skill in contrived scenarios. Should the learner struggle to use the skill independently, the interventionist may first use a gestural prompt. This may take the form of pointing to their eyes and mouth, indicating that the learner may look to those areas for clues about how someone is feeling. If the individual successfully used the skill following the gestural prompt, no additional prompts would be provided. If unsuccessful skill use was observed, the next level of prompt (e.g., written or verbal) would be provided to the learner.

Visual or Activity Schedules

Visual or activity schedules describe a type of antecedent intervention in which an individual is provided with a sequential description of a skill or task to be completed, with the description provided often using a combination of pictures and written text. This strategy is intended to build upon visual skills of individuals with ASD (e.g., Janzen, 2003), presenting information in a manner that may be more meaningful and impactful (Schneider & Goldstein, 2010). Further, visual or activity schedules have been suggested as being helpful in reducing anxiety about activities, providing learners with more concrete information and expectations about what may occur.

Visual or activity schedules are prepared in a manner similar to a task analysis. That is, a complex task or activity is broken down into smaller, discrete steps. For each step, a picture or icon that represents that step, sometimes with corresponding text, is prepared. Visual schedules are typically prepared in a format that is portable (e.g., on a clipboard), allowing the learner to transport the schedule to the relevant setting and reference it as needed.

Once prepared, the visual or activity schedule would then be presented to the learner prior to the time at which the skill or social activity is expected to occur. An interventionist may present the visual or activity schedule with instructions such as "let's see what you need to do" (Daneshvar et al., 2019, p. 3). The learner may then be introduced to the setting in which the behavior is expected to be demonstrated, with the visual schedule continuing to be available to the learner to reference as they complete the skill or activity. As a learner demonstrates each step within the schedule, they may mark it as complete (e.g., checking off an item, moving a picture to a "complete" column). If necessary, an interventionist may provide prompts to the learner to reference the activity schedule should they need support—with prompts to reference the schedule being reduced as the learner demonstrates increased independence in demonstrating the skill or activity sequence.

Environmental Modifications

Environmental modifications describe procedures in which contextual variables would be altered as a means of prompting use of a social skill, with no direct training or support in the actual skill itself. In making modifications to the environment, interventionists should aim to decrease the response effort required to demonstrate target skills and reduce barriers that may prevent skill use from occurring.

In order to effectively implement environmental modifications, it is first critical to identify environmental features that may facilitate or hinder social skill use. For this reason, a comprehensive and cross-environment assessment may be critical to identifying elements that may support learners with ASD. Once identified, barriers to skill use may be removed and facilitators of skill use may be introduced. This may take the form of introducing preferred activities and stimuli of the learner with ASD into a social environment (e.g., preferred game), bringing the learner with ASD and peers into closer proximity and providing increased opportunities for interaction and use of social skills. Relatedly, environmental modification may employ creation of activities that require coordinated efforts among individuals—again, increasing the opportunities for social interaction and engagement. Simultaneously to these modifications, interventionists may consider removing distracting or aversive stimuli from the environment as a means of increasing approach behaviors of learners with ASD to social situations.

Advantages of Antecedent Interventions

As described above, a wide range of antecedent social skills teaching strategies may be considered to support learners with ASD. Although procedural variations exist across the aforementioned strategies, all procedures have the potential to impact a behavior prior to its occurrence. Social skills teaching strategies that rely on consequent interventions (e.g., provision of positive reinforcement) would allow a learner to demonstrate less effective social skills before receiving feedback on more effective skill use. This may be somewhat inefficient, as a learner may require a substantial number of opportunities for consequences in order to acquire a target skill.

Antecedent strategies, however, aim to prevent less effective social skill use from occurring. That is, individuals are provided with support prior to a skill being used, increasing the likelihood that a more effective variation of a social skill is demonstrated during each opportunity to use a skill. This may ultimately benefit the learner in acquiring and generalizing skill use due to frequent contact with reinforcement provided for more effective skill use. Overall, antecedent interventions represent a proactive model of intervention, setting up learners to encounter frequent positive reinforcement for more effective social skill use.

Empirical Basis

The literature base investigating antecedent strategies to promote social skills performance deficits is robust and generally supports them as effective for this purpose. For example, the National Standards Project (National Autism Center, 2015) identified two antecedent interventions that were classified as established treatments according to project criteria, schedules and antecedent components of broader behavioral intervention strategies (e.g., prompting, auditory scripting). Although the NSP (2015) describes schedules as effective for promoting self-regulation skills, which may be relevant to social interaction but are not social behaviors as defined in this text, others have used scripting to directly impact specific social skills. For example, Budzińska et al. (2014) created an activity schedule for a 3-year-old child with ASD that included six components of a structured social interaction between the child and their teacher. The components included (1) selecting an activity, (2) approaching the classroom teacher, (3) attending to the teacher, (4) requesting initiation of the activity with the teacher, (5) waiting for the teacher's response, and (6) participating in the activity. The authors found that this activity schedule, in combination with another antecedent strategy (i.e., the provision of scripts), led to increases in unprompted social initiations by the child as well as generalization of responding to novel adults.

The NSP's (2015) classification of other antecedent strategies as established treatments part of a larger behavioral intervention package is reflective of their flexibility and frequent use alongside other effective strategies; however, there is evidence to support these additional antecedent strategies as effective when they are isolated from other components. In fact, Ledford et al. (2018) identified prompting as "the most frequently used stand-alone antecedent intervention" (p. 8) and there are numerous examples of its use in the literature. For example, Kinsella et al. (2017) developed software to be used with Google Glass technology that would monitor conversational speech within the wearer's environment and provide a range of response suggestions to the wearer as prompts for appropriate social interaction. Once the Google Glass detected a response by the wearer, it would resume monitoring for conversational speech in anticipation of the next prompt. While wearing this device, all ten participating children with ASD were able to navigate a ten-turn conversational exchange in a simulated restaurant-themed scenario with a research assistant.

A more traditional example of stand-alone prompting was conducted by Charlop-Christy and Kelso (2003). They used cue cards, which, despite their name, functioned as prompts rather than cues due to their intrusive nature within the social environment. In this study, children with ASD were engaged in conversations by the researchers and immediately presented a card with a scripted response and a prompt to "read it." The researchers also examined presentation of the cards following a 10 s time delay as well as a testing period in which no prompts were provided at all. They found that correct social responding during the conversations with researchers increased when the cue cards were used and maintained during the no-card testing period. Further, they found that correct social responding generalized to different topics and conversational partners, suggesting that the children were not prompt dependent and could generalize conversational skills to novel settings.

In addition to the NSP's (2015) endorsement of antecedent strategies as effective, a recent synthesis of this literature revealed additional experimental support. Ledford et al. (2018) conducted a meta-analysis and identified a number of antecedent interventions as effective based on their success rate (i.e., the percentage of studies examining each strategy that documented consistent positive effects on participants' social skills). Specifically, they identified prompting, prompting plus scripting, modification of environmental arrangements, and prompting plus modification of environmental arrangements as effective strategies, each with a success rate of 89% or higher. Each of these success rates were based on an accumulation of single-case experimental design evidence (i.e., greater than ten studies per strategy). Similarly, Radley et al. (2020) identified a range of antecedent strategies (i.e., prompting, schedules, physical space modification, and activity modification) as commonly used to address social skill deficits in individuals with ASD. Although they did not perform a quantitative synthesis of the literature, they noted that nearly 80% of studies examining antecedent interventions met the What Works Clearinghouse single-case design standards (Kratochwill et al., 2010), suggesting the supporting evidence was of high quality and scientifically rigorous.

Both syntheses also provide insight into which learner, setting, or outcome variables may be important to consider before deciding to implement an antecedent strategy. The Ledford et al. (2018) meta-analysis examined learner age, interventionist, and social partner to determine if any of these contributed to differential success rates across the various antecedent strategies. They found that prompting alone was slightly more effective for older learners (i.e., 11 and older) than it was for younger learners (i.e., <11) whereas the reverse was true for prompting plus scripting. Modification of environmental arrangements with and without a prompting component was only ever examined in learners younger than 11 but was found to be highly effective for this population. Regarding the implementer or interventionist, only prompting demonstrated robust success rates across researchers, teachers, and other interventionists (e.g., parents or peers). Prompting with scripting and prompting with environmental modifications was effective across researcher and teacher implementation while environmental modifications alone was only ever investigated with the researcher as interventionists. Thus, when considering antecedent interventions to address social skills deficits in individuals with ASD across a wide range of interventionists, prompting procedures may be the best strategy. Finally, an examination of the social partner selected for the intervention process reveals one interesting detail. Prompting alone and combined with a scripting component was less effective when the researcher acted as the social partner than when others acted as the social partner. The other antecedent strategies were equally effective across social partners; however, choosing individuals from the learner's natural environment (i.e., not researchers) may be desirable to promote generalization of performance outside of the teaching environment.

Radley et al. (2020) review also examined the age of participants included in antecedent intervention studies as well as the particular outcome targeted by the interventions. Consistent with Ledford et al. (2018) review, they found that the majority of this literature targeted younger learners with an average participant age of 8.4 years; however, a wide age range was identified (range = 3–21 years). This average age is consistent with other antecedent strategies involving direct training for skill acquisition (i.e., BST and video modeling). When considering the outcomes addressed by antecedent strategies, Radley et al. (2020) found that social engagement was targeted twice as often as social skill accuracy, which makes sense given its utility as a performance deficit strategy rather than an acquisition deficits strategy. What follows next is a brief review of the literature supporting antecedent interventions to promote social behavior in individuals with ASD. The studies selected for this review were chosen due to the range of utility they capture and do not necessarily represent a comprehensive view of this literature. Readers are directed to the two syntheses referenced above for more detailed reviews.

Empirical Examples

First, Tzanakaki et al. (2014) investigated the use of tactile prompts to increase social initiations made by five children with ASD toward their typically developing peers in free play settings. In this study, children were taught to ask a question to a therapist every time a prompting device (i.e., Motviaider, 2017) vibrated on the table in front of them. It was set to vibrate every 30 s. Therapists used a most-to-least prompting procedure until each child was able to independently ask questions to the examiner when the device vibrated. Additionally, children were given rule cards with examples of questions they might ask of the therapist during the teaching procedure. Once training was complete, the children were sent into a 10 min free play session with typically developing peers while keeping the tactile prompting device in their pocket, this time set to vibrate on 1-min intervals. If a child exhibited ten social initiations (i.e., one for each prompt) they were able to earn a preferred reinforcer. The researchers found that this procedure was very effective in promoting social initiations above pre-treatment levels and in a follow-up study found that the tactile prompts could be gradually faded.

In another example, Betz et al. (2008) used joint activity schedules to promote social engagement between preschoolers with ASD and their typically developing peers. In this study, the researchers created photographic activity schedules containing two preselected games and four additional games from which children could choose two. The participants with ASD were paired with one of their typically developing peers for the duration of the study and these dyads were responsible for working through the activity schedule. Each page of the activity schedule had a picture of one of the dyad members, indicating which member was responsible for which page. Included on the pages were scripts to prompt participants to interact with one another (e.g., "Let's play…"). The researchers estimated the duration of social engagement between dyad members as well as the number of prompts required to facilitate engagement between the two. With the activity schedule in place, participants and their peers were observed to engage in a large amount of social interaction, much higher than pre-treatment levels. Further, the number of prompts required by the researchers steadily declined over subsequent sessions with the schedule in place. The researchers eventually faded their presence out of the intervention and demonstrated consistently high levels of engagement but did not examine whether those levels maintained in the absence of the activity schedule.

Finally, Caballero and Connell (2010) examined the effectiveness of social cue cards on the social communication skills of three preschool students with diagnoses of ASD. Participants' social interaction with same-aged peers was observed during 30 min free play sessions. For each participant, a set of social cue cards were developed which specified a social behavior, the relevant antecedent stimuli for performing that behavior, and an identified positive reinforcer for exhibiting the behavior. Researchers reviewed the cards prior to each session with each participant and conducted a comprehension assessment for each card, asking WH-questions related to each card's content. Then, if participants exhibited any of the behaviors detailed by their social cue cards during a free play session, researchers immediately provided them access to the specified reinforcer. This procedure resulted in uniform increases in social skills across the three participants and these increases were maintained after a fading procedure was conducted in which the frequency of the social cue card review was reduced to once or twice each week. Additionally, participants were observed to exhibit the targeted social behaviors in settings in which the social cue cards were not present, suggesting the performance increases generalized.

Practical Case Example

To highlight the practical utility of antecedent interventions and provide additional examples of how they may be used to address deficits in social skills, three case examples are described below for prompting, social schedules, and modification of the physical environment.

Prompting Ethan is a 10-year-old child with ASD whose caregiver report is having difficulty interacting with peers in public and community settings (e.g., library story hour, community parks). They report that he does not attempt to initiate social interactions with other children his age yet frequently expresses a desire to make friends and play with others in these settings. Through an interview and some direct skills assessment you determine that Ethan knows how to initiate conversations on topics he is interested in as well as invite others to join in ongoing games or activities. Working from the hypothesis that the social skill deficit is performance-based, you decide to recommend a prompting intervention that can be implemented by Ethan's parents when they are present with him in these settings.

Together with Ethan and his caregiver, you develop a prompting procedure that involves the caregiver observing Ethan and verbally prompting him to initiate conversations with peers (or invite them to join his play) every 5 min so long as he is not socially engaged at that time. This procedure will require his caregiver to observe him briefly every 5 min to determine his engagement status and if not engaged, approach and provide a brief verbal prompt. Because Ethan reported difficulty thinking of what to say in the moment, his caregiver will also provide one example of what he could say to initiate a conversation. You encourage his caregiver to track the number of 5 min intervals that Ethan is not engaged with peers in these settings for 1 week before beginning the prompting procedure and continuing to collect these data upon implementation in order to assess its effectiveness. Additionally, in order to incentivize Ethan to initiate social interaction without the need for a prompt, his caregiver will keep track of the number of 5 min intervals without a prompt and award Ethan one point for each. His caregiver agrees to develop a menu of reinforcing activities and stimuli for which he can exchange his points.

Social Schedule Abigail is a 4-year-old child with ASD whose teacher reports is not interacting with peers during free play time in her pre-Kindergarten classroom. During this time, students are free to select one of several center activities (e.g., costume play, building, art) and engage in appropriate social play with classroom peers. Abigail has been observed to sit in her chair in a corner of the room and not engage with any of the center activities nor her peers; however, during aftercare when Abigail is in the room with fewer peers she is observed moving about the classroom and engaging with many different activity centers. Because of this, Abigail's teacher believes her behavior during free play time is due to difficulty navigating the classroom in the presence of peers and decides that a social schedule may provide her with the additional support needed to be successful in this environment.

Abigail's teacher creates a schedule for her that contains pictures of each of the five activity centers. Each picture is placed on a separate sheet of paper and the five papers are stapled together to create a small social schedule booklet. At the top of every page is the name of the center as well as smaller pictures of ways in which students can interact in the centers. Abigail's teacher has planned to meet briefly with Abigail 5-min prior to the start of free play time each day and review the social schedule booklet. She also informs Abigail that she would like her to try to engage each of the centers in the order in which they appear in the book and that every 5 min she will check on her to ask if she would like to continue at her current center or switch to the next center. During these meetings she will also give Abigail ideas for how she might interact appropriately with her peers at each center and ask Abigail to list her own ideas as well.

Modification of Physical Space or Activities Finn is a 15-year-old adolescent with ASD who was referred by his English teacher for being isolated from peers. The teacher noted that during group activities, Finn is frequently observed to work by himself. Although peers may invite Finn to join their group, he is often unresponsive to initiations from peers. Finn's teacher reports that they have observed Finn engage with peers about particular topics (e.g., video games), and that he does seem to have social skills that would allow him to effectively join in groups and engage with peers. As it appears that Finn has the requisite skills to be able to engage with peers during group activities, you recommend that his teacher implement environmental modifications that may facilitate Finn's engagement.

Finn's teacher identifies that students in their class will be completing a group assignment in which a group will complete a "news broadcast," creating a headline, writing a script, planning a broadcast, and filming the broadcast for presentation in the class. You recommend that the teacher modify the assignment to incorporate Finn's interests. Specifically, you suggest that the teacher assign groups a topic, with Finn's group being assigned the topic of video games. The teacher agrees that this may be helpful to engage Finn in the project, and his teacher incorporates this into their lesson plan. In class, Finn's teacher presents the assignment to the class and assigns Finn's group to develop a news broadcast on video games. Finn's teacher observes him to be notably more engaged with his peers. Finn volunteers to be the newscaster in the videotaped broadcast, which is particularly noteworthy as Finn has previously declined to do in-class presentations. Finn's teacher considers the antecedent strategy to be a success. They chat with Finn about other topics that may be of interest to him in group projects and plan to incorporate those topics into future group assignments.

Conclusion

To summarize, antecedent strategies as described here do not explicitly teach specific social behavior but instead serve to prompt learners to exhibit social skills, provide visual aids for learners to reference, or structure environments in ways that make appropriate social interaction less effortful or aversive. These strategies are typically more effective in remediating performance, rather than acquisition, deficits in elementary school aged children (e.g., 6–11). Although they may be implemented in isolation, antecedent interventions are often combined with other components such as reinforcement contingencies or explicit instruction in order to maximize their effectiveness. Practitioners should consider implementing antecedent interventions when they wish to increase the frequency of social behaviors or duration of social engagement within a naturalistic environment.

References

Betz, A., Higbee, T. S., & Reagon, K. A. (2008). Using joint activity schedules to promote peer engagement in preschoolers with autism. *Journal of Applied Behavior Analysis, 41*, 237–241.

Budzińska, A., Lubomirska, A., Wójcik, M., Krantz, P. J., & McClannahan, L. (2014). Use of scripts and script-fading procedures and activity schedules to develop spontaneous social interaction in a three-year-old girl with autism. *Health Psychology Report, 2*, 67–71.

Caballero, A., & Connell, J. E. (2010). Evaluation of the effects of social cue cards for preschool age children with autism spectrum disorders (ASD). *Journal of Behavior Assessment and Intervention in Children, 1*, 25–42.

Charlop-Christy, M. H., & Kelso, S. E. (2003). Teaching children with autism conversational speech using a cue card/written script program. *Education and Treatment of Children, 26*, 108–127.

Cooper, J. O., Heron, T. E., & Heward, W. L. (2020). *Applied behavior analysis*. Pearson.

Daneshvar, S. D., Charlop, M. H., & Malmberg, D. B. (2019). A treatment comparison study of a photo activity schedule and Social Stories for teaching social skills to children with Autism Spectrum Disorder: Brief report. *Developmental Neurorehabilitation, 22*, 209–214.

Janzen, J. E. (2003). *Understanding the nature of autism: A guide to the autism spectrum disorders* (2nd ed.). Communication Skill Builders.

Kinsella, B. G., Chow, S., & Kushki, A. (2017). Evaluating the usability of a wearable social skills training technology for children with autism spectrum disorder. *Frontiers in Robotics and AI, 4*, 1–31.

Kratochwill, T. R., Hitchcock, J., Horner, R. H., Levin, J. R., Odom, S. L., Rindskopf, D. M & Shadish, W. R. (2010). *Single-case designs technical documentation*. Retrieved from What Works Clearinghouse website: http://ies.ed.gov/ncee/wwc/pdf/wwc_scd.pdf.

Ledford, J. R., King, S., Harbin, E. R., & Zimmerman, K. N. (2018). Antecedent social skills interventions for individuals with ASD: What works, for whom, and under what conditions? *Focus on Autism and Other Developmental Disabilities, 33*, 3–13.

Mayer, G., Sulzer-Azaroff, B., & Wallace, M. (2012). *Behavior analysis for lasting change* (2nd ed.). Sloan Publishing, LLC.

MotivAider. (2017). *MotivAider®: Making people better, one habit at a time*. (Behavioral Dynamics) Retrieved from http://habitchange.com/

Moxley, R. A. (1996). The import of Skinner's three-term contingency. *Behavior and Philosophy, 24*, 145–167.

National Autism Center. (2015). *Findings and conclusions: National standards project, Phase 2*. Retrieved from http://www.nationalautismcenter.org/

Radley, K. C., & Dart, E. H. (2016). Antecedent strategies to promote children's and adolescents' compliance with adult requests: A review of the literature. *Clinical Child and Family Psychology Review, 19*, 39–54.

Radley, K. C., Dart, E. H., Brennan, K. J., Helbig, K. A., Lehman, E. L., Silberman, M., & Mendanhall, K. (2020). Social skills teaching for individuals with autism spectrum disorder: A systematic review. *Advances in Neurodevelopmental Disorders, 4*, 215–226.

Schneider, N., & Goldstein, H. (2010). Using social stories and visual schedules to improve socially appropriate behaviors in children with autism. *Journal of Positive Behavior Interventions, 12*, 149–160.

Tzanakaki, P., Grindle, C. F., Dungait, S., Hulson-Jones, A., Saville, M., Hughes, J. C., & Hastings, R. P. (2014). Use of a tactile prompt to increase social initiations in children with autism. *Research in Autism Spectrum Disorders, 8*, 726–736.

Waters, M. B., Lerman, D. C., & Hovanetz, A. N. (2009). Separate and combined effects of visual schedules and extinction plus differential reinforcement on problem behavior occasioned by transitions. *Journal of Applied Behavior Analysis, 42*, 309–313.

Chapter 8
Manualized Social Skills Curricula

Manualized social skills curricula is a term that describes social skills teaching interventions that are prepared by someone other than the intended end user, resulting in a social skills curricula that is pre-packaged and ready for implementation. Although manualized social skills curricula may vary in the individual components they include, most include lesson plans and other intervention materials that allow a practitioner to avoid having to independently develop intervention materials for use in social skills curricula. Other elements commonly observed in manualized curricula include task analysis of target skills, ready-made progress monitoring tools, and reinforcement strategies to increase learner engagement. All together, the elements of manualized social skills curricula primarily serve to decrease interventionist demand in facilitating social skills teaching, increase integrity of implementation, augment data-based decision making, and potentially speed the transition of research to practice.

As previously stated, a defining characteristic of manualized social skills curricula is that they are composed of pre-packaged intervention materials. Interventions may vary in the degree of practice-readiness of the manualized intervention, with some interventions providing general guidelines for implementation (e.g., outline for social skills teaching that can be applied to skills of the facilitators selection), whereas others provide detailed, step-by-step teaching plans for each skill to be taught and provide a facilitator with all needed materials. Regardless of where a curriculum is along this continuum, manualized curricula serve to decrease the demand placed on a facilitator to develop and implement social skills teaching. Specifically, manualized social skill curricula eliminate the need for a facilitator to independently develop and implement all elements of an intervention through provision of intervention supports (e.g., Radley et al., 2014a, b). Ultimately, the pre-packaged nature of manualized social skills curricula reduces barriers to implementation such as lack of resources, training required for implementation, or

K. C Radley, E. H. Dart, *Social Skills Teaching for Individuals with Autism*, Springer Series on Child and Family Studies,
https://doi.org/10.1007/978-3-030-91665-7_8

availability of technology that may limit facilitator adoption of non-manualized social skills teaching strategies (e.g., Bellini & McConnell, 2010).

In addition to reducing facilitator demand related to development and implementation of social skills teaching, manualized social skills curricula likely serve to increase fidelity of implementation of intervention. Fidelity of implementation is critical to determining whether an intervention was beneficial (e.g., Gresham et al., 2000). Many manualized social skills curricula provide step-by-step guides to implementation, which may limit implementation drift over time. Given the tightly structured nature of manualized social skills curricula, facilitators may therefore be able to more closely approximate implementation of social skills teaching in research contexts—increasing the likelihood that similar outcomes may be observed.

Many manualized social skill curricula incorporate assessment materials as part of the curriculum. This may consist of formative assessments that provide the facilitator with guidance regarding skills to be taught or baseline levels of social skill use. Assessment that is built into manualized social skill curricula may also be summative. For example, a curriculum may provide a facilitator with progress monitoring tools to gauge learner progress toward goals and determine the need for reteaching. Curricula may also provide assessment that links learner progress to other outcomes (e.g., individualized education plan goals).

Previous social skills research has indicated that evidence-based social skills teaching strategies may be underused in applied contexts (e.g., Stahmer, 2007). For example, Hess et al. (2008) found that facilitators often implemented unsupported social skills teaching strategies in school settings. Dingfelder and Mandell (2011) suggested that interventions that lack an accompanying curriculum as a delivery vehicle may experience barriers to adoption. Therefore, manualized social skills curricula that incorporate evidence-based practices may aid in bridging the research-to-practice gap. However, as not all manualized social skill curricula incorporate evidence-based practices, it remains critical that practitioners are able to identify evidence-based social skills teaching strategies.

Although use of manualized social skills curricula is associated with the previously described benefits, limitations of manualized social skills curricula should also be noted. Primarily, manualized social skill curricula may be inflexible to learner needs. Because manualized curricula typically come with pre-made lesson plans, facilitators are limited to teaching those skills already described within the curriculum. For example, the PEERS for Young Adults (Laugeson, 2017) manual contains 17 lessons—any skill not described within those 17 lessons would therefore be unaddressed by the program. Because of their inflexible nature, it is therefore unlikely that any one social skills curriculum would meet the needs of all individuals; thus, it behooves the facilitator to select a curriculum that most closely matches the needs of individuals receiving social skills teaching.

A second limitation of manualized social skill curricula is the potential cost of the curriculum. Compared to social skills teaching strategies which rely on facilitator-created materials to implement, most manualized social skill curricula are commercially published. Thus, facilitators are unable to recreate the intervention themselves and would be required to purchase the curriculum in order to implement it. Whereas some curricula are comprised only of a treatment manual and may therefore be relatively inexpensive, other curricula may involve multiple components (e.g., manual, videos, reward materials) and represent a substantial investment in intervention materials. To illustrate, at the time of publication, the Peers for Young Adults curriculum (manual only) retailed for $69.95, whereas the Superheroes Social Skills curriculum (manual, videos, associated intervention materials) retailed for $865.00. The high cost of some intervention curricula may therefore represent a barrier to use in applied contexts.

Manualized Curricula Composition

Manualized social skills curricula vary in terms of skills taught and active intervention elements. Most, however, share some basic features that are intended to promote acquisition and use of target social skills. Specifically, many manualized curricula will incorporate some or all elements of behavioral skills training (BST), in which a description of skill steps is provided, a model is viewed, learners have the opportunity to rehearse the skill, and feedback is provided regarding skill use. As described in Chap. 4, BST represents an empirically supported social skills teaching practice and may increase the likelihood that a manualized intervention results in favorable outcomes. Whereas BST is incorporated into many manualized curricula, other empirically supported strategies discussed in this text are also incorporated to a lesser extent. For example, Superheroes Social Skills (Jenson et al., 2011) incorporates video models (Chap. 3), peer-mediated intervention (Chap. 6), and self-management (Chap. 9), and LEGO Club includes peer-mediated components. The incorporation of multiple evidence-based strategies has been suggested to support acquisition and generalization of skills (e.g., Radley et al., 2014a, b; Sofronoff et al., 2017), though such a practice may unnecessarily introduce additional, unneeded, intervention components (Radley et al., 2021).

Whereas BST typically serves as a critical, empirically supported ingredient in manualized social skills curricula, interventionists are also advised to select curricula with other essential social skills teaching elements. Krasny et al. (2003) describe nine critical principles that should be incorporated into social skills curricula. Although not an exhaustive list of best practices in social skills teaching, Krasny et al. suggest social skills curricula should aim to make the abstract concrete, provide structure and predictability, provided scaffolded language support, provide multiple and varied learning opportunities, include "other"-focused activities, foster self-awareness and self-esteem, set relevant goals, program in a sequential and graded manner, and provide opportunities for programmed generalization and ongoing practice.

Krasny et al. (2003) suggest that curricula should aim to make abstract social skills more concrete through explicitly operationalizing social behaviors, facilitating differentiation between occurrences and non-occurrences of target social skills. Manualized curricula that incorporate task analyses of social skills, breaking skills down into smaller, discrete steps, meet this standard. Curricula may also use visual cues and other prompts that facilitate understanding and use of skills. Structure and predictability may be demonstrated in manualized curricula that utilize consistent lesson plans, teaching social skills in a similar manner across lessons. Other examples of structure and predictability may include lessons that begin and end in a consistent manner (e.g., similar opening activity). Scaffolded language in manualized curricula is incorporated through grouping learners by language ability, ensuring that all learners in a group are able to benefit from instruction. For learners that require additional support, visual cues may be provided to facilitate acquisition and generalization of skills. Krasny et al. also suggest that curricula should incorporate multiple and diverse learning opportunities (e.g., Stokes & Baer, 1977). Curricula that incorporate multiple evidence-based strategies (e.g., video modeling, BST) provide learners with diverse opportunities to learn and practice target skills, increasing the likelihood that skills are generalized to non-training environments.

Krasny et al. (2003) propose that social skills curricula should focus on the social nature of social skills. That is, skills that are meant to be used in a pair or group setting should not be practiced with a learner in isolation. Further, a focus on others may promote recognition that use of social skills can be enjoyable and beneficial to learners. Self-awareness and self-esteem should be incorporated into curricula by setting up environments that result in high levels of reinforcement for social skill use, focus on strengths and interests of learners, and celebrate individuality of learners. In setting relevant goals, practitioners utilizing social skills curricula should prioritize skills that are most relevant to a learner. That is, any one particular manualized social skill curricula may or may not adequately meet the social needs of a learner or group of learners. Prioritizing critical skills may also be accomplished through providing rationale in skill instruction, highlighting why a particular skill may be important or relevant for use. Related to goals, programming should be sequential and graded—simplifying complex skills into more discrete behaviors and organizing instruction such that later lessons build upon previous lessons. Finally, Krasny et al. emphasize that curricula should plan for generalization through provision of learning opportunities across settings (e.g., home, school), such that instruction and practice does not occur in one isolated setting. Other strategies that curricula may incorporate consist of including peers in social skills groups and providing homework activities.

Example Manualized Social Skill Curricula

A substantial number of manualized social skill curricula are available to practitioners. For example, Gaffney (2020) identified over 40 curricula that are commercially available to practitioners to teach social skills to learners with ASD. As such, a review of all available curricula and their accompanying empirical support is beyond the scope of this chapter. However, several widely utilized or researched curricula will be reviewed to provide examples of elements that practitioners may encounter when selecting a manualized social skills curriculum.

Program for Education and Enrichment of Personal Skills (PEERS)

PEERS (Laugeson & Frankel, 2010) is a widely used and available social skills curriculum for adolescents with ASD. PEERS lessons follow a predictable format, with social skills teaching occurring over 14 90-min lessons presented once per week. PEERS is taught in a group format, with each lesson focusing on a discrete social skill. During each PEERS lesson, learners review previous homework, receive didactic instruction in a target social skill, view models of the skill, role-play the skill, receive feedback regarding skill use, and are given a new homework assignment. Lessons in the PEERS manual are intended to be taught sequentially, and lessons not meant to be skipped. Parents or caregivers of learners play a pivotal role in PEERS, helping learners complete assignments outside of lessons. Included in the curriculum are program-specific assessments that may be used to determine response to intervention. Since publication of the initial PEERS curriculum, several extensions of the program have been published and are available to practitioners. Specifically, a school-based manual (Laugeson, 2014) and a manual for adults with ASD (Laugeson, 2017) have been published, with other variations also being investigated (e.g., preschool-age learners, PEERS for dating).

Superheroes Social Skills

Superheroes Social Skills (Jenson et al., 2011) is a multimedia social skills curriculum developed for elementary-age learners with ASD. A total of 17 social skills are taught within the program, with skills ordered from foundational to advanced. Superheroes Social Skills is unique in that much of the instruction is delivered via video-based animated superhero characters. As previously described, Superheroes Social Skills incorporates multiple evidence-based practices, including BST, video modeling, and self-management of skill use. Similar to PEERS, Superheroes Social Skills lessons all share a similar format. At the start of each lesson, the facilitator checks in with learners and reviews homework from previous lessons. A lesson schedule is then reviewed and the facilitator introduces a target social skill, describing a rationale for skill use. Next, participants are provided with a self-management card to track skill use during group, as well as out of group. Learners then view a video in which an animated superhero describes the discrete steps to demonstrating the target skill. Following, learners view videos of unknown peers demonstrating the skill. Next, the facilitator models skill use and engages learners in role-play of the skill—providing performance feedback throughout. Participants then view an animated social narrative in which a superhero character uses the skill, followed by participation in a social game that requires use of the target skill. During both the role-plays and social game, participants are encouraged to monitor skill use on the self-management card. At the conclusion of each group, learners are provided with homework and receive reinforcement for participation in the group. Similar to PEERS, the Superheroes Social Skills manual contains program-specific assessments that may be used to monitor progress.

Skillstreaming

Skillstreaming (McGinnis & Goldstein, 1984) is social skills curriculum that teaches social skills using a BST format. Several iterations of the curriculum are available, with one being specific to social needs of learners with ASD and related disorders. Within the manual, skills are grouped into six areas: relationship skills, social comprehension, self-regulation, problem-solving, understanding emotions, and school-related skills, with a total of 80 different social skills being taught within the curriculum. Each lesson follows a similar format, with discrete steps to skill use being defined at the beginning of each lesson. Learners then discuss rationale for skill use, see a model of skill use, participate in guided practice, and receive feedback. Skillstreaming also programs for generalization through identifying skill practice in other, non-training settings, as a critical element of lessons. Reproducible homework forms are included for each skill taught, and included checklists can be used to evaluate social skill use.

Lego® Club

Relative to the three previously described curricula, LEGO Club (Legoff et al., 2010) represents a somewhat less structured social skills curriculum. That is, specific target social skills are not explicitly task analyzed and taught. Instead, LEGO Club aims to promote social skills by setting up opportunities to participate in social interactions using a commonly preferred medium (i.e., LEGOs). During each LEGO Club session, learners are greeted and assigned one of three roles: engineer, supplier, or builder. Learners then work together to build a lego model, engaging in problem-solving and communication in order to complete the model. Learners are then provided with unstructured time to play with LEGO, allowing for further use and refinement of social skills. The LEGO Club intervention incorporates a behavior management system, providing learners with rewards for demonstrating group expectations.

Empirical Basis

The literature supporting manualized curricula for addressing social skills deficits in individuals with ASD is robust. A systematic review of single-case research by Radley et al. (2020) identified this strategy as one of the most popular, with 24 studies reporting the results of empirical investigations of manualized social skills curricula. The participants in those studies were typically between 7 and 8 years old although the range spanned ages 3 through 18. Further, the outcomes assessed in those studies were evenly split between social skill accuracy and social skill engagement, reinforcing the idea that manualized curricula are suitable for addressing both acquisition and performance deficits.

Although there are many systematic reviews and meta-analyses synthesizing the social skill treatment literature, few isolate the effects of manualized curricula, making it difficult to determine if this general strategy is more or less effective relative to other broad strategies (e.g., video modeling). For example, Gates et al. (2017) conducted a meta-analysis of group-based social skills interventions for individuals with ASD and found that they were generally effective ($g = 0.51$). Manualized social skills curricula are often delivered in a group-based format and this synthesis included investigations of manualized programs (i.e., *SkillStreaming*; Lopata et al., 2010); however, non-manualized programs (e.g., peer networking; Kamps et al., 2015) were also included. Although Gates et al. (2017) did examine some moderators of treatment effect (e.g., informant) but whether the group-based social skill intervention incorporated the use of a manualized curriculum was not systematically examined.

Despite this limitation of the broader social skills teaching literature base, there are many individual studies and some program-specific syntheses to support certain manualized social skills teaching programs (e.g., the PEERS curriculum). Thus, the remainder of this section will present brief reviews of the evidence supporting some of the most popular curricula.

PEERS In one of the first experimental investigations of the PEERS curriculum, Laugeson et al. (2009) demonstrated its effectiveness with a large group of adolescents (ages 13–17) with ASD. They found that implementation of PEERS over 12 weeks resulted in increases in adolescents' reports of social interaction with peers, knowledge of appropriate social interaction, and friendship quality. Parent reports of their adolescents' social behavior also increased following completion of the treatment; however, participants' teacher reports did not reflect substantial therapeutic change, suggesting treatment effects were limited to home and community settings. In a follow-up study, Laugeson et al. (2012) again examined PEERS' effectiveness on adolescents' social interaction, knowledge of social skills, and friendship quality but also extended the investigation to include an assessment of its durability over time, or maintenance. In this study, the PEERS curriculum was implemented over a 14-week period and participants' responsiveness was assessed; however, an additional 14-week follow-up assessment was also administered to participants to determine whether the initial effects of the PEERS curriculum were maintained over time. Laugeson et al. (2012) found that nearly all of the treatment effects evident following the 14-week implementation of PEERS remained evident following the 14-week follow-up period. These data suggest that the PEERS curriculum not only teaches appropriate social behavior to individuals but may also promote performance of these behaviors in naturalistic settings.

Mandelberg and colleagues (2014) conducted a very long-term evaluation of the effects of PEERS and found that improvements on standardized measures of social skill performance (i.e., the Social Responsiveness Scale and Social Skills Rating System) were maintained through a 5-year follow-up period following implementation of the PEERS curriculum. Matthews et al. (2018) extended these initial investigations of PEERS by examining its impact on other related outcomes, such as adolescent well-being, loneliness, and social anxiety. In their investigation, Matthews et al. (2018) found that PEERS not only increased social skill knowledge but also had positive impacts on self-reported loneliness and social anxiety.

Further, the primary effects of PEERS have been replicated across many different research teams (e.g., Radley et al., 2018) and settings (e.g., Japan; Yamada et al., 2020), suggesting its effectiveness is not tied to specific clinicians or populations other than those with ASD. A recent meta-analysis of nine PEERS studies (Zheng et al., 2021) identified the largest treatment effects for social knowledge and moderate effects on parent-report of social functioning. Finally, McVey et al. (2017) examined whether gender differences in clients predicted differential treatment effects with PEERS and found that both males and females with ASD exhibited similar responses to treatment. In sum, the evidence supporting PEERS as an effective manualized curriculum to support individuals with ASD in their social skill acquisition and performance is overwhelmingly positive.

Superheroes Social Skills The evidence supporting Superheroes Social Skills is plentiful, but differs from the PEERS evidence in two important ways. First, whereas PEERS studies almost exclusively use group experimental designs to evaluate its effectiveness, the Superheroes Social Skills literature exclusively uses single-case experimental design. Second, PEERS evaluations rely heavily on standardized indirect assessment of social outcomes (e.g., rating scales) whereas evaluations of Superheroes Social Skills rely primarily on direct measure of social behavior (e.g., direct observation). Neither of these differences substantially alter the strength of the evidence supporting either strategy; however, measurement choices within social skills teaching paradigms (described in more detail in Chap. 2) may influence the extent to which clinicians can attribute implementation of a treatment to changes in clients' social behavior.

The first empirical evaluation of Superheroes Social Skills was published by Radley et al. (2014a) and aimed to investigate its feasibility when used within a parent training model. Two previous unpublished investigations (i.e., Block, 2010; Hood, 2010) had established its effectiveness as a manualized program implemented by researchers. Radley and colleagues (2014a, b) found that parents were able to implement the Superheroes program with integrity across an 8-week period and improvements in social initiations, social responses, and total social engagement were observed for most participants. Follow-up studies have replicated these findings with researchers serving as the clinicians but have extended them in meaningful ways.

For example, Radley et al. (2014b) implemented an 8-week Superheroes Social Skills curriculum with three elementary school students (ages 8–10) with ASD to evaluate whether the effects generalized to a novel setting (i.e., playground during recess). Not only did they find participants engaging in increased social engagement, initiations, and responses with peers throughout the program's implementation, they identified an effect on some participants' social standing. Specifically, using an index of social salience, they found that two participants were identified as less marginalized by their peers and more centrally located within peer groups. These data provide insight into the indirect effects of social skills teaching and the positive impacts of such programs. In a more recent study, Radley et al. (2021) conducted a component analysis of the Superheroes Social Skills program and found that the largest social skill acquisition and accuracy benefits for participants were observed during sessions in which all program components were implemented. These findings suggest that manualized curricula may not confer maximal benefit when components of the programs are not implemented or modified in some way.

Skillstreaming Unlike PEERS and Superheroes Social Skills, Skillstreaming was not developed specifically for individuals with ASD; however, it is one of the most well-established social skills treatment manuals (Goldstein et al., 1980) and there have been several investigations of its use specifically with individuals with ASD and it remains popular for this purpose. Lopata et al. (2010) evaluated the effectiveness of Skillstreaming on parental report of their child's social functioning related to features of ASD. Notably, the sample of children (7–12 years old; $M = 9.39$) were all considered "high-functioning" with average or above average cognitive profiles. Skillstreaming was implemented with participants 1 day each week for 5 weeks and each day consisted of five treatment cycles. Treatment cycles were each 70 min and consisted of a 20-min Skillstreaming instructional period followed by a 50-min therapeutic activity where social skills could be practiced. Thus, participants received nearly 6 h of treatment activities once per week with nearly two of those hours dedicated solely to Skillstreaming instruction. Although intensive, improvements were observed on nearly all parent-completed rating scales and direct assessments of participants' behavior including those involving emotion recognition, complex language use, and social knowledge.

More recently, Lerner and Mikami (2012) compared Skillstreaming to another social skills program called Sociodramatic Affective Relational Intervention (SDARI). The two were compared because of the differences between their theoretical mechanisms with Skillstreaming being classified as knowledge-based and SDARI being classified as performance-based. These classifications describe each by their primary mode of instruction with Skillstreaming using components of BST to promote skill acquisition through direct instruction (i.e., knowledge) and SDARI using structured games and activities where success relies on performance of social behavior. The children participants in this study were slightly older ($M = 11.33$) but were not necessarily "higher-functioning" as in the Lopata et al. (2010) study. Lerner and Mikami (2012) found that while SDARI conferred immediate benefits to participants' social interaction and peer liking after one session, these gains were ultimately reversed over the 10-week course of treatment; however, participants in the Skillstreaming group demonstrated steady and long-term growth in peer liking and social interaction. Both groups improved on staff-reported social skills. Thus, there is evidence to suggest that the structured, knowledge-based approach found in Skillstreaming (and many other manualized curricula) may be more effective than those based in other treatment modalities.

Lego® Club Social skills interventions involving Lego® have a surprisingly large supporting literature base given their central focus on a popular toy brick. A review of Lego® therapy to improve social functioning in individuals with ASD was conducted by Lindsay et al. (2017) who identified 15 articles meeting their search criteria. Across these 15 studies, they identified a large amount of variability in treatment session formats (i.e., 20–90 min, once weekly, anywhere from 4 weeks to 3 years). This is not entirely unexpected because unlike the other manualized curricula, which specify specific lesson sequences and durations, Lego® Club is performance-based (like SDARI described above) and play sessions can continue indefinitely once the group structure is established. Further, they reported that the individual responsible for arranging the Lego® Club within each study also varied based on their relationship to the participants (e.g., researcher, parent) and qualifications. Lindsay et al. (2017) noted that of the 15 included studies, nearly all (i.e., 14) reported improvement on at least one outcome, supporting its effectiveness.

Other studies have investigated the short- and long-term outcomes of Lego® Club interventions on children and adolescents' social functioning. For example, Owens et al. (2008) found that immediate improvements in social interaction were attributable to participation in a Lego® Club program and these improvements outperformed those observed in a different treatment group. Legoff and Sherman (2006) found that participants in a Lego® Club intervention demonstrated improved adaptive behavior and social interaction 3 years later, suggesting the skills learned during Lego® Club activities maintained over time. As with Skillstreaming, it is not uncommon to see children with average or above average intelligence and language ability participate in Lego® Club rather than other treatment modalities due to its less structured setting and heavy reliance on peer-to-peer interaction. To highlight its flexibility, Levy and Dunsmuir (2020) arranged Lego® Club groups to be implemented by school staff in a secondary setting (i.e., high school). They recruited six adolescents with ASD to participate in a twice weekly group lasting 45 min across a 6-week intervention period. Levy and Dunsmuir (2020) documented increases in students' social interaction, social initiation, and social responses as a result of their participation in the group.

Generalization

As with any social skills teaching package, generalization of skills beyond the teaching setting is an important consideration (see Chap. 12); however, it may be most important when using manualized curricula due to the fact that they are often implemented in extremely contrived settings (e.g., clinic, therapy room). DuPaul and Eckert (1994) reviewed seven studies using manualized curricula to teach social skills with an emphasis on the generalization of their effects. They found mixed results, noting that generalization of skills was minimal when researchers failed to use intentional generalization strategies and more effective when a combination of strategies were used. Although detailed and specific generalization strategies will be discussed in Chap. 12, McIntosh and MacKay (2008) make several recommendations to make social skills curricula effective once the lesson concludes including: use an incentive system to promote performance in the generalization setting, have learners use self-monitoring to track their performance, move lessons to naturalistic settings, involve others, increase opportunities for practice, and choose skills that are used frequently. Although not exhaustive, this list provides clinicians with a small example of the strategies that might be considered to ensure that learners are exhibiting learned skills across environments. It is critical that clinicians not assume learners will generalize learned skills from the teaching setting to other settings. Failing to plan for generalization into other settings besides the manualized treatment group setting will likely not result in socially significant behavior change.

Practical Case Example

Dr. O'Ryan is a psychologist who facilitates a weekly social skills group for 11- and 12-year-old individuals with ASD. Dr. O'Ryan is beginning a new group, and is seeking to determine which skills would be most beneficial for group members. In order to do so, Dr. O'Ryan distributes a social skills checklist to parents and guardians of group participants. Once completed and returned, Dr. O'Ryan reviews the checklists to determine commonly identified concerns. She then makes a list of all possible social skills that may benefit from teaching and compares this list to skills taught within extant social skills curricula. In doing so, she determines that the skills align with those taught within the Superheroes Social Skills program—in particular, the skills from the foundational and intermediate skills section of the program.

Dr. O'Ryan decides to work sequentially through the two sections of the Superheroes Social Skills program, given that these skills were endorsed as needs for nearly all participants in the group. Each social skill lesson from the program is taught in a weekly group. Dr. O'Ryan follows the manual for each lesson, with each lesson following an identical format of presentation of a target skill, video models of skills, roleplay and feedback, and additional opportunities to view models and practice the target skill. During each lesson, Dr. O'Ryan takes data regarding skill acquisition of group members. When all members of the group are able to demonstrate target skills with 100% accuracy, Dr. O'Ryan introduces a new target skill.

This procedure is repeated until all skills from the foundational and intermediate skills sections of the Superheroes Social Skills program have been taught. At the end of the intervention, Dr. O'Ryan distributes the same checklist to parents and guardians in order to determine changes in perceptions of skill use. Across participants, ratings generally indicate perceived improvements on behalf of parents and guardians—indicating greater skill use in generalized contexts. Given these data, Dr. O'Ryan determines that the group has been effective in addressing initial concerns noted across group members.

Conclusion

To summarize, manualized social skills curricula are useful, and may be preferable, to those clinicians who would prefer a more structured (but somewhat less flexible) treatment option that requires less intervention development than many of the other strategies described in this text. Although many of these curricula are knowledge-based, meaning they primarily address acquisition deficits, some (e.g., Lego® Club) are performance-based and are more suited to address performance-deficits. In either case, it is important to consider the cognitive and language abilities of your clients when selecting a manualized curriculum as many incorporate a great deal of verbal-mediation compared to more behavioral treatments. Finally, it is paramount that clinicians using manualized social skills curricula incorporate plans for their learners to generalize skill performance across settings.

References

Bellini, S., & McConnell, L. L. (2010). Strength-based educational programming for students with autism spectrum disorders: A case for video self-modeling. *Preventing School Failure: Alternative Education for Children and Youth, 54*, 220–227.

Block, H. (2010). *"Superhero social skills": A pilot study examining an evidence-based program for elementary-aged students with autism spectrum disorders in a school setting*. Unpublished doctoral dissertation, University of Utah.

Dingfelder, H. E., & Mandell, D. S. (2011). Bridging the research-to-practice gap in autism intervention: An application of diffusion of innovation theory. *Journal of Autism and Developmental Disorders, 41*, 597–609.

DuPaul, G. J., & Eckert, T. L. (1994). The effects of social skills curricula: Now you see them, now you don't. *School Psychology Quarterly, 9*, 113–132.

Gaffney, A. M. (2020, January). *Social skills curriculum for individuals on the autism spectrum*. Indiana Resource Center for Autism. https://www.iidc.indiana.edu/irca/articles/assets/social-skills-curriculum-2020.pdf

Gates, J. A., Kang, E., & Lerner, M. D. (2017). Efficacy of group social skills interventions for youth with autism spectrum disorder: A systematic review and meta-analysis. *Clinical Psychology Review, 52*, 164–181.

Goldstein, A. P., Sprafkin, R. P., Gershaw, N. J., & Klein, P. (1980). *Skillstreaming the adolescent.* Research Press Company.

Gresham, F. M., MacMillan, D. L., Beebe-Frankenberger, M. E., & Bocian, K. M. (2000). Treatment integrity in learning disabilities intervention research: Do we really know how treatments are implemented? *Learning Disabilities Research & Practice, 15*, 198–205.

Hess, K. L., Morrier, M. J., Heflin, L. J., & Ivey, M. L. (2008). Autism treatment survey: Services received by children with autism spectrum disorders in public school classrooms. *Journal of Autism and Developmental Disorders, 38*, 961–971.

Hood, J. (2010). *Is "Superheroes Social Skills" an evidence-based approach to teach social skills to children in a clinical setting? A pilot study examining an evidence-basedprogram for children with autism.* Unpublished doctoral dissertation, University of Utah.

Jenson, W. R., Bowen, J., Clark, E., Block, H., Gabriensen, T., Hood, J., Radley, K. C., & Springer, B. (2011). *Superheroes social skills*. Ancora Publishing.

Kamps, D., Thiemann-Bourque, K., Heitzman-Powell, L., Schwartz, I., Rosenberg, N., Mason, R., & Cox, S. (2015). A comprehensive peer network intervention to improve social communication of children with autism spectrum disorders: A randomized trial in kindergarten and first grade. *Journal of Autism and Developmental Disorders, 45*, 1809–1824.

Krasny, L., Williams, B. J., Provencal, S., & Ozonoff, S. (2003). Social skills interventions for the autism spectrum: Essential ingredients and a model curriculum. *Child and Adolescent Psychiatric Clinics, 12*, 107–122.

Laugeson, E. (2017). *PEERS® for young adults: Social skills training for adults with autism spectrum disorder and other social challenges*. Routledge.

Laugeson, E. A. (2014). *The PEERS curriculum for school based professionals: Social skills training for adolescents with autism spectrum disorder*. Routledge.

Laugeson, E. A., & Frankel, F. (2010). *Social skills for teenagers with developmental and autism spectrum disorders: The PEERS Treatment Manual*. Routledge.

Laugeson, E. A., Frankel, F., Gantman, A., Dillon, A. R., & Mogil, C. (2012). Evidence-based social skills training for adolescents with autism spectrum disorders: The UCLA PEERS program. *Journal of Autism and Developmental Disorders, 42*, 1025–1036.

Laugeson, E. A., Frankel, F., Mogil, C., & Dillon, A. R. (2009). Parent-assisted social skills training to improve friendships in teens with autism spectrum disorders. *Journal of Autism and Developmental Disorders, 39*, 596–606.

Legoff, D. B., Krauss, G. W., & Levin, S. A. (2010). LEGO®-based play therapy for autistic spectrum children. In A. A. Drewes & C. E. Schaefer (Eds.), *School-based play therapy* (2nd ed., pp. 221–235). John Wiley & Sons.

Legoff, D. B., & Sherman, M. (2006). Long-term outcome of social skills intervention based on interactive LEGO© play. *Autism, 10*, 317–329.

Lerner, M. D., & Mikami, A. Y. (2012). A preliminary randomized controlled trial of two social skills interventions for youth with high-functioning autism spectrum disorders. *Focus on Autism and Other Developmental Disabilities, 27*, 147–157.

Levy, J., & Dunsmuir, S. (2020). Lego therapy: Building social skills for adolescents with an autism spectrum disorder. *Educational and Child Psychology, 37*, 58–83.

Lindsay, S., Hounsell, K. G., & Cassiani, C. (2017). A scoping review of the role of LEGO® therapy for improving inclusion and social skills among children and youth with autism. *Disability and Health Journal, 10*, 173–182.

Lopata, C., Thomeer, M. L., Volker, M. A., Toomey, J. A., Nida, R. E., Lee, G. K., & Rodgers, J. D. (2010). RCT of a manualized social treatment for high-functioning autism spectrum disorders. *Journal of Autism and Developmental Disorders, 40*, 1297–1310.

Mandelberg, J., Laugeson, E. A., Cunningham, T. D., Ellingsen, R., Bates, S., & Frankel, F. (2014). Long-term treatment outcomes for parent-assisted social skills training for adolescents with autism spectrum disorders: The UCLA PEERS program. *Journal of Mental Health Research in Intellectual Disabilities, 7*, 45–73.

Matthews, N. L., Orr, B. C., Warriner, K., DeCarlo, M., Sorensen, M., Laflin, J., & Smith, C. J. (2018). Exploring the effectiveness of a peer-mediated model of the PEERS curriculum: A pilot randomized control trial. *Journal of Autism and Developmental Disorders, 48*, 2458–2475.

McGinnis, E., & Goldstein, A. P. (1984). *Skillstreaming the elementary school child*. Research Press Company.

McIntosh, K., & MacKay, L. D. (2008). Enhancing generalization of social skills: Making social skills curricula effective after the lesson. *Beyond Behavior, 18*(1), 18–25.

McVey, A. J., Schiltz, H., Haendel, A., Dolan, B. K., Willar, K. S., Pleiss, S., Karst, J. S., Carson, A. M., Caiozzo, C., Vogt, E., & Van Hecke, A. V. (2017). Brief report: Does gender matter in intervention for ASD? Examining the impact of the PEERS® social skills intervention on social behavior among females with ASD. *Journal of Autism and Developmental Disorders, 47*, 2282–2289.

Owens, G., Granader, Y., Humphrey, A., & Baron-Cohen, S. (2008). LEGO® therapy and the social use of language programme: An evaluation of two social skills interventions for children with high functioning autism and Asperger syndrome. *Journal of Autism and Developmental Disorders, 38*, 1944–1957.

Radley, K. C., Dart, E. H., Brennan, K. J., Helbig, K. A., Lehman, E. L., Silberman, M., & Mendanhall, K. (2020). Social skills teaching for individuals with autism spectrum disorder: A systematic review. *Advances in Neurodevelopmental Disorders, 4*, 215–226.

Radley, K. C., Ford, W. B., Battaglia, A. A., & McHugh, M. B. (2014b). The effects of a social skills training package on social engagement of children with autism spectrum disorders in a generalized recess setting. *Focus on Autism and Other Developmental Disabilities, 29*, 216–229.

Radley, K. C., Helbig, K. A., Murphy, A. N., McCargo, M. G., & Lown, E. L. (2018). The effects of a modified PEERS curriculum on accurate and novel responding of children with autism spectrum disorder. *Advances in Neurodevelopmental Disorders, 2*, 412–424.

Radley, K. C., Helbig, K. A., Schrieber, S. R., Ware, M. E., & Dart, E. H. (2021). Superheroes social skills: A comparison of video only and full curriculum on social skill use. *Focus on Autism and Other Developmental Disabilities, 36*, 95–107.

Radley, K. C., Jenson, W. R., Clark, E., & O'Neill, R. E. (2014a). The feasibility and effects of a parent-facilitated social skills training program on social engagement of children with autism spectrum disorders. *Psychology in the Schools, 51*, 241–255.

Sofronoff, K., Silva, J., & Beaumont, R. (2017). The secret agent society social-emotional skills program for children with a high-functioning autism spectrum disorder: A parent-directed trial. *Focus on Autism and Other Developmental Disabilities, 32*, 55–70.

Stahmer, A. C. (2007). The basic structure of community early intervention programs for children with autism: Provider descriptions. *Journal of Autism and Developmental Disorders, 37*, 1344–1354.

Stokes, T. F., & Baer, D. M. (1977). An implicit technology of generalization. *Journal of Applied Behavior Analysis, 10*, 349–367.

Yamada, T., Miura, Y., Oi, M., Akatsuka, N., Tanaka, K., Tsukidate, N., Yamamoto, T., Okuno, H., Nakashi, M., Taniike, M., Mohri, I., & Laugeson, E. A. (2020). Examining the treatment efficacy of PEERS in Japan: Improving social skills among adolescents with Autism Spectrum Disorder. *Journal of Autism and Developmental Disorders, 50*, 976–997.

Zheng, S., Kim, H., Salzman, E., Ankenman, K., & Bent, S. (2021). Improving social knowledge and skills among adolescents with autism: Systematic review and meta-analysis of UCLA PEERS® for adolescents. *Journal of Autism and Developmental Disorders, 51*(12), 4488–4503.

Chapter 9
Self-Management

Self-management refers to three distinct processes through which a learner is taught to engage in some form of assessment of their own behavior, make a determination about whether their behavior is aligned with environmental or social expectations, and deliver a consequence based on that determination. The first process, self-monitoring, involves assessment of the target behavior by the learner. For example, a learner may be asked to count the number of times they initiate social interaction with a peer during a specific time of the day. The second process, self-evaluation, refers to the comparison of the self-assessment to some criterion or goal. For example, a learner may be asked to determine whether the number of social initiations they exhibited exceeded their goal of ten for the day. Finally, self-reinforcement refers to the consequential component, whereby a learner might provide themselves access to some reinforcing stimulus (e.g., a new book) if their performance met or exceeded the criterion.

Self-management may be best conceptualized as the behavioral component of self-regulation, a broader concept that "subsumes the regulation not only of behavior but also of thoughts and emotions" (Inzlicht et al., 2021, p. 321). The link between self-regulation and social competence is strong. For example, McKown et al. (2009) found parent- and teacher-report of child self-regulation to be a strong predictor of social competence across two studies, one of typically developing children and one of children referred to a psychological clinic. Further, a review by Eisenberg et al. (2010) identified a link between effortful control (i.e., self-regulation) and social competence both in children and adults. For individuals with ASD, who often present with deficits in social competence, these findings suggest that the deficits may stem from difficulties in self-regulation. Although they are not part of the DSM diagnostic criteria, some have suggested that "the neurobiology of autism increases the vulnerability to the development of self-regulation difficulties, resulting in an area of significant clinical concern for many individuals with autism of different ages and functioning levels" (Hepburn & Wolff, 2013, p. 429). Thus, it

K. C Radley, E. H. Dart, *Social Skills Teaching for Individuals with Autism*,
Springer Series on Child and Family Studies,
https://doi.org/10.1007/978-3-030-91665-7_9

is plausible that individuals with ASD are more likely to experience difficulties in self-regulation, leading to lower social competence and poorer quality of social interactions. Self-management is an appealing treatment strategy due to its focus on structuring self-regulation processes for specific target behaviors based on the needs of the learner; however, because it does not explicitly teach skills it should be thought of exclusively as a strategy to remediate performance deficits unless it is combined with teaching procedures (e.g., behavioral skills training; Chap. 4).

One of the earliest treatment evaluations of self-management on participants' social behavior was conducted by Zegiob et al. (1978), who found that two individuals with intellectual disability were able to reduce their own socially undesirable behavior simply by self-recording it over an extended period of time (i.e., self-monitoring), despite their poor accuracy in doing so. Treatments incorporating self-management may use one, two, or all three processes, depending on the needs and capability of the learner. In any case, behavior change under a self-management procedure is often called reactivity, as it is thought to be a result of the learner's reaction to one of the three processes. There are several theoretical explanations for why this reactivity may occur.

Nelson and Hayes (1981) summarize three alternative explanations for why self-management procedures lead to behavior change. First, they describe Kanfer's (1977) three-stage model of self-regulation, which posits that the self-administered contingencies present in the self-reinforcement processes are sufficient to generate motivation in the learner to modify their behavior to meet the criterion for reinforcement. Next, they introduce Rachlin's (1974) explanation, which states that self-monitoring, self-evaluation, and self-reinforcement serve as signals to the individual that there are more distal environmental consequences outside of the self-monitoring process and it is these contingencies that ultimately drive increases or decreases in responding. Finally, Nelson and Hayes (1981) extend Rachlin's (1974) explanation by adding that it is a collection of environmental stimuli, not just the learner's reactivity to the self-management processes, that signal the availability of more distal consequences. That is, they posit that it is the presence of the environmental cues (e.g., recording devices, individuals involved in training) and self-management that signal to the learner the availability of other environmental contingencies. Although not inconsistent with each other, these three theories offer sequentially more complete explanations for how self-management comes to exert change in a learner's behavior.

The following three subsections of this chapter will each examine one of the three sub-processes of self-management more closely, providing a description of their essential elements and considerations for practice.

Self-Monitoring The first self-management process, self-monitoring, involves teaching an individual to make a record of the target behavior as it occurs. To do this, it is necessary first to identify the behavior to be monitored. As mentioned in Chap. 2, target behaviors should be operationally defined, with clear and precise language and specifying examples and non-examples. This will allow the learner to make more consistent decisions about whether they engaged in the target behavior or not by reducing ambiguity about its occurrence. Further, target behaviors should be socially significant and appropriate targets for change. Whether the goal is for the learner to increase the frequency of a desirable social behavior or decrease the frequency of an undesirable social behavior, the appropriateness of the goal should be considered by the teacher as well as any other stakeholders (including the learner) involved in the behavior change process.

Next, it is necessary to determine the method by which the learner will conduct their assessments. Perhaps most common is a simple frequency count. That is, the learner would record a tally mark for every time they observe themselves exhibiting the behavior. This method of measurement would be most useful when the target behavior is discrete and not multi-step. For example, a frequency count might be appropriate when self-monitoring social initiations taking the form of a question (e.g., "How are you today?"). A learner could easily count the number of times they asked a question of another individual that was not part of an ongoing social exchange. Other continuous recording assessment methods that may be useful in self-monitoring include duration, latency, and intensity. For example, a learner may be asked to keep a record of the total duration of social interaction between themselves and any other individuals in their immediate environment. Doing so would be more effortful than a frequency count but would provide a more complete picture of the learner's total social engagement across a monitoring period than a frequency count of social initiations would.

In addition to continuous recording (e.g., frequency counts), learners may be given the option to self-monitor their behavior using discontinuous measurement methods (e.g., interval recording; Cooper et al., 2020); however, these methods are more complex and would require more training than may be possible. In that case, rating scales or hybrid behavior assessment methods (i.e., direct behavior ratings; e.g., Smith et al., 2018) represent an acceptable alternative. Learners could be asked to complete a rating to estimate the frequency or duration with which they exhibited a behavior over some period of time. These could be repeated somewhat frequently, allowing the learner to generate multiple estimates of their behavior over a short period of time. Further, rating scales might allow learners to measure additional dimensions of their behavior such as quality. For example, a learner might be asked to rate the overall quality of their social interactions each hour on a 10-point scale or make a single summative rating of quality. In either case, the learner would need to be taught the elements of high-quality social interaction before being asked to make these judgments and the scale would need to reflect stepwise increases in quality.

Regardless of which measurement method is selected, keep in mind that all are associated with at least some material components. Frequency counts require paper and a writing utensil, but can also be taken using electronic devices (e.g., smartphones, tablets) or tokens. Duration recording and the discontinuous measurement methods all require the learner to keep track of time using a stopwatch or other electronic device. Rating scales may be completed on paper using a writing utensil or digitally with an electronic device and survey tools (e.g., Qualtrics). Select the measurement method that is most suitable for the behavior of interest but consider whether the material requirements of that method do not create a burden on the learner by reducing their ability to participate in their environment while monitoring is taking place.

The final component of self-monitoring involves the identification of a schedule and whether any self-monitoring cues are needed. The schedule can be derived from the learner's specific needs. For example, if the goal is to increase social interaction in a large group setting at school (e.g., recess), then the monitoring period would be limited to that specific setting. The learner would be asked to perform a self-monitoring assessment of their social interaction each school day during recess. If the learner is expected to conduct multiple self-assessments throughout the monitoring period, consider adding a prompt to their environment for them to conduct the assessment at regular intervals. This could be a reminder from the teacher or other individual in their environment, a tactile prompt from an electronic device such as a Motivaider (2017), or some other environmental stimulus change such as a light changing colors or turning on, a brief noise or tone, or a tap on the shoulder. The learner should be aware of what these prompts mean prior to beginning the self-monitoring process.

Self-Evaluation As mentioned previously, self-monitoring is just the first of three distinct self-management processes. The second, self-evaluation, refers to how the learner processes the data that were collected during the self-monitoring process. Self-evaluation requires the learner to compare their performance against a pre-established criterion. This criterion functions as a goal for performance and should be set by the teacher prior to self-evaluation. The goals set for learners should be empirically derived, meaning they are based on data and not generated arbitrarily. For example, you may observe that typically developing peers on a playground setting exhibit between five and ten social initiations per hour. This figure could be used to set a goal for a learner's social initiations in the same setting. Keep in mind that performance expectations may change across settings, communities, and cultures and that goals should be developed with those expectations and relevant data on hand. In other words, it would not be appropriate to always expect learners to exhibit between five and ten social initiations per hour. The environmental context and cultural expectations may modify what is considered appropriate. Initial self-evaluation goals may be set lower than a terminal goal if the learner's performance is not expected to rise rapidly. Doing so would also provide the learner with early achievement within the self-management process and increase the likelihood that they continue to engage.

When engaging in self-evaluation, learners are asked simply to compare the data they collected during self-monitoring to their performance goal. Thus, it is critical that the goal selected for evaluation matches the form of the data being collected. That is, it would not be appropriate to select a goal of "80% or more of social initiation task analysis steps exhibited, on average" when the learner is self-monitoring the frequency of social initiations. Also, it is sometimes desirable to increase a learner's goals, particularly when initial goals are set relatively low to encourage participation and success. Just like the initial goal setting process, modified goals should be based on incoming data to ensure that they are not set too lofty or too low. Teachers are encouraged to use a method such as percentile shaping (e.g., Galbicka, 1994) to incrementally increase self-evaluation goals as learners have success with initial goals.

Additional elements can be added to the self-evaluation process to increase the saliency of the learner's performance. For example, it is not uncommon to have learners keep a chart or graph of their performance. Learners may be asked to maintain a running graph of their performance over days or weeks and plot each data point following every self-monitoring session. This form of self-evaluation could be used to track performance over a longer period of time rather than session-to-session performance. Other stimuli can be used to make goals more salient to learners during the self-monitoring process. For example, teachers, when prompting self-monitoring, may also provide a learner with a reminder of their goal for the day (e.g., "It's time to self-monitor and remember, your goal for today is seven social initiations"). Alternatively, this reminder could be a printed numerical goal on the learner's self-monitoring form on which they are recording their data. The self-evaluation process could also include a way for learners to indicate that their goal was met such as a check box or a shape for them to fill in if they determine that their goal was met.

Self-Reinforcement The final self-management process, self-reinforcement, is relatively simple and often occurs hand-in-hand with self-evaluation. If a learner, through self-evaluation, determines that they have met their goal, then self-reinforcement would have them deliver a reinforcing consequence to themselves for doing so. It is this reinforcement process that, in part along with more distal natural contingencies, drives changes in behavior within the self-management process. When establishing a self-reinforcement process, it is important to identify reinforcing stimuli that the learner can access and deliver themselves to maintain autonomy throughout the process. For reinforcing stimuli that are less easily deliverable (e.g., activity-based) it may be desirable to establish a token economy (e.g., Shapiro et al., 1980; Reinecke et al., 1999) to provide learners with immediate access to backup reinforcers after each successful self-evaluation period that can later be exchanged for primary reinforcers.

Another concern often described throughout the self-management process but particularly during self-reinforcement is the issue of learner accuracy. When the monitoring, evaluation, and reinforcement process is turned over entirely to the learner one wonders whether the process is being conducted accurately. That is, learners may intentionally or unintentionally commit errors in monitoring which lead to errors in evaluation and errors in reinforcement. When this happens, learners may contact reinforcement for a change in behavior that did not occur, circumventing the intervention process. To address this concern, it is not uncommon for teachers to keep separate records of learner behavior using the exact same monitoring system, creating an independent but identical record to which the learner's self-monitoring record can be compared. Although it is more effortful on the teacher, the ability to verify the learner's record eliminates the possibility of inadvertent reinforcement. Additionally, it may be helpful to set initial goals based only on accuracy between the learner and teacher at first rather than changes in frequency or duration of the target behavior. This process could serve to build rapport and understanding between the teacher and learner while giving the teacher confidence that the learner can self-monitor accurately and giving the learner opportunities to receive feedback on their records.

Teaching Self-Management

Although relatively straightforward, the self-management process can vary in many ways (e.g., target behavior, measurement, frequency, goal setting) and learners should never be expected to take on the task without sufficient training in the processes and procedures. Teachers should engage learners in a behavioral skills training (BST) package aimed at increasing their understanding and accuracy of the specific self-management program developed for their needs. Recall that BST includes didactic instruction, modeling, roleplay, and feedback to maximize learning and opportunities for practice. When using self-management, ensure that learners have demonstrated mastery of the processes within a BST environment before expecting them to implement them in naturalistic settings.

Advantages

Two of the most obvious benefits of self-management programs are their portability and the extent to which they promote generalization and maintenance of skill performance. Because learners are primarily responsible for engaging in self-management processes with minimal involvement from others, they are easier than other intervention strategies to transfer between settings. Because of this, the treatment effects of self-management are also more likely to generalize across settings. Stokes and Osnes (1989) explain that interventions using self-mediated physical, verbal, and covert stimuli are more likely to produce generalizable effects. Self-management uses stimuli such as prompts, self-monitoring recording materials, and the learner's public and private verbalizations to mediate treatment effects across settings, making it ideal from a generalization perspective. Peterson et al. (1999) provided a demonstration of this phenomenon, using self-management to promote generalization of social skills acquisition to non-training classroom settings in 29 middle school students at-risk for developing behavioral disorders.

Additional benefits of self-management include its low intensity relative to other teaching strategies (e.g., social skills groups, peer-mediated strategies) and lessened effort on the teacher to maintain over time; however, recall that self-management is a performance-deficit intervention, meaning it cannot be used to address skill acquisition without modifications or additional components. Thus, although it is low intensity, its scope is limited to cases in which learners have already acquired the targeted social skills but have not yet begun to perform them in naturalistic settings.

Empirical Basis of Self-Management

As previously described, self-management represents an intervention strategy that has frequently been used to teach social skills. Subsequently, multiple summaries of research have included self-management interventions within their analyses. These summaries have generally supported self-management as an empirically supported social skills teaching strategy.

In reviewing literature published between 1957 and 2012, the National Autism Center (2015) identified 31 studies that had utilized self-management as an intervention strategy for individuals with ASD. Self-management was identified as an Established Intervention, though it should be noted that not all of the identified 31 studies targeted social outcomes. Of note, however, is that one-third of intervention research in self-management took place between 2007 and 2012, suggesting an increase in the use of the procedure within research contexts.

Whereas the National Standards Project (2015) does not provide a quantitative metric of the effect of self-management interventions for individuals with ASD, other researchers have endeavored to do so. In one example, Lee et al. (2007) meta-analyzed social skills teaching interventions for individuals with ASD published between 1992 and 2001. A total of 11 articles were identified for inclusion, with a total of 34 participants included across the studies. The majority of these studies were conducted in school settings, and although the meta-analysis was not limited to only social outcomes, social outcomes were assessed in 25 of the 34 participants. Overall analysis of the data indicated that self-management studies represented an effective teaching strategy for individuals with ASD. Considering social outcomes, results suggested that self-management interventions were more effective for non-social behaviors—although the authors reported that differences in effect size between social and non-social behaviors were not statistically significant.

Carr et al. (2014) provide an additional meta-analysis of self-management interventions, including research published prior to November 2012. A total of 29 studies were identified for inclusion, with 70 participants being included in these studies. Similar to Lee et al. (2007), identification of studies was not limited to only those with social outcomes. However, social skills were assessed in the majority of participants (70%). Again, self-management was identified as an effective social skills teaching strategy for individuals with ASD—though the calculated effect size suggested that self-management was less effective for social skills than it was for academic skills and activities of daily living. Other findings of the meta-analysis indicate that self-management may be effectively utilized with school-age individuals through adulthood, with individuals of varying levels of cognitive functioning, and across a variety of settings (e.g., home, community, clinic).

Whereas Carr et al. (2014) did not code self-management research as taking place in school settings, Davis et al. (2016) conducted a meta-analysis of self-management interventions only conducted in school settings. Articles published between 1960 and 2014 were considered for inclusion, with 16 studies identified that included a total of 28 participants. The overall effect size was identified to represent a strong effect (Tau-U = 0.83) though this analysis was not limited to only social outcomes. Unlike previous meta-analyses, social outcomes were not identified as the most frequently assessed; however, social outcomes were found to have relatively stronger effects compared to other outcomes assessed. As with Carr et al. (2014), who found self-management to only produce questionable effects for very young children with ASD, Davis et al. indicated that effects were most notable for elementary and secondary students with ASD. Whereas as other researchers had documented the general effectiveness of self-management across settings (e.g., home, school), Davis et al. found self-management to be effective across settings within a school (e.g., self-contained, general education)—further highlighting the utility of self-management for school-based professionals. An additional meta-analysis has further indicated the general effectiveness of self-management procedures in inclusive settings (Watkins et al., 2019).

In a systematic review of literature published between 1998 and 2018, Radley et al. (2020) identified eight studies that utilized self-management interventions as a social skills teaching intervention. These studies included 18 participants, who were an average of 8 years old. Most of the studies identified assessed social skill accuracy, with fewer assessing outcomes such as social engagement and ratings of social functioning. All of the studies identified in the review met What Works Clearinghouse standards with or without reservations with respect to methodological quality.

Taken together, the various meta-analyses and systematic reviews indicate that self-management strategies represent an empirically supported social skills teaching strategy for individuals with ASD. However, extant data suggest that self-management may not be universally effective for all learners with ASD—particularly for those younger than elementary school-age. Further, it should be emphasized that relatively few meta-analyses have focused exclusively on self-management for social skills. Despite this, meta-analyses that have considered social functioning as an outcome variable have documented the effectiveness of self-management—despite some studies suggesting that other outcomes (e.g., activities of daily living; Carr et al., 2014) are more amenable to self-management interventions.

Implementation Examples from the Literature

Examples of self-management interventions consist of the use of self-management in isolation, as well as in conjunction with other teaching strategies. Koegel et al. (1992) provide an early example of self-management being utilized in isolation from other social skills teaching strategies. As part of the study, four children with ASD who demonstrated unresponsiveness to the initiations of others were recruited for participation. All participants were of elementary school-age. Intervention consisted of teaching participants to use a wrist counter to track response to initiations of others. Initially, participants were taught to discriminate between occurrences and non-occurrences of the target behavior, thus allowing for accurate self-monitoring. Participants were provided with a reward after demonstrating accurate self-monitoring, with the number of instances of accurate self-management being required for reinforcement increasing over time. Whereas self-management was initially introduced in a clinic setting, it was eventually introduced to community, home, and school settings. Results of the study indicated that self-management was initially successful with three of four participants, with one participant requiring additional training to reduce variability in responding. Equally important, participants demonstrated improvements in responding not only in the training setting, but also in generalized settings. Data also suggested that participants were highly accurate in use of self-management procedures, and that reductions in disruptive behavior were observed as a collateral effect of self-management of responses to initiations.

Liu et al. (2015) also demonstrated the utility of self-management in isolation from other social skills teaching procedures. A single participant, a 9-year-old girl with ASD, was included in the study. She was reported to have a comorbid intellectual disability, engage in destructive behavior, and have delays in both expressive and receptive language. Lui et al. used video recordings of target behaviors in training discrimination between occurrences and non-occurrences of social behaviors—consisting of no interruption, asking for opinions, and appropriately greeting unfamiliar adults. Discrimination training consisted of viewing videos and asking the participant whether the behavior demonstrated was appropriate or inappropriate, and continuing until the participant was able to respond correctly to all questions. At this point, the researchers conducted self-monitoring training, with self-monitoring accomplished by the participant coloring a picture of a flower following each occurrence of a target behavior. During intervention, verbal praise was provided following each demonstration of the appropriate behavior, and edible reinforcers (i.e., chocolate bars) were initially provided on a fixed ratio schedule. Implementation of the self-management intervention resulted in large and immediate increases in the use of target behaviors. Once initial increases were obtained, self-management was faded from implementation, with increases in target skill use being observed at 1-month follow-up. Further, changes in target social skill use were observed to generalize across persons—further suggesting the utility of self-management procedures for social skills teaching.

Parker and Kamps (2011) also implemented self-management, but instead of tracking general skill performance, the two participants with ASD self-monitored discrete steps to completion of three different social activities. Peers were included in the study, and provided prompts and opportunities for the participants with ASD to demonstrate social skill use. Implementation of self-management was found to result in large and rapid increases in the number of social activity steps for two of three activities, with smaller increases observed for the third skill. Other data collected indicated that activity engagement increased during the intervention phase, as did peer-directed verbalizations.

Just as self-management has been evaluated in isolation from other social skills teaching strategies, it has also been investigated as part of multi-component social skills teaching interventions. Hood et al. (2020) implemented social skills teaching using behavioral skills training for three individuals with ASD. Participants in the study first engaged in behavioral skills training (see Chap. 4) as a means of teaching skills related to giving and accepting compliments. Whereas this was sufficient for most participants, one participant demonstrated variability in responding for one skill. As a result, self-management was introduced in addition to BST. The addition of self-management consisted of the participant engaging in discrimination training and then engaging in self-monitoring of accurate skill use. Following the addition of self-management, immediate increases in skill use were observed.

In another multi-component intervention, Apple et al. (2005) evaluated the effects of video modeling in isolation and in conjunction with self-monitoring on compliment giving of children with ASD. Three-, four-, and five-year-old participants engaged in video modeling for initiating and responding to compliments. All participants demonstrated initial increases following video modeling. Next, video modeling was discontinued and self-management introduced as a means of promoting maintenance of skills. Results of the study indicated that the inclusion of self-management procedures resulted in continued use of skills learned without the need for external monitoring. That is, participants were able to maintain improvements in target skills with minimal additional support (e.g., reinforcement) required. The authors describe these results as demonstration of the ability of self-management to increase independence, serving as a pivotal behavior in learning, generalizing, and monitoring a range of other behaviors.

Guide to Practice

Implementation of a self-management intervention, as with any social skills teaching strategy, must begin with identifying and operationally defining behavioral targets. Clear definitions are critical and will support other steps to implementation (e.g., discrimination training). In developing operational definitions, practitioners should focus on using specific definitions instead of vague descriptions of behavior. As such, it would be preferable to define a target as "responds to peers initiations within 10-s" instead of something less specific (e.g., "shows good friendship").

When teaching multi-step skills, practitioners should develop a task analysis of the skill (e.g., Parker & Kamps, 2011)—allowing learners to engage in self-management across all steps of a skill. For example, the skill of exiting a conversation could be monitored across discrete steps to the skill. This could entail steps such as waiting for a pause in the conversation, providing a reason for leaving or ending the conversation, and saying goodbye.

Next, practitioners must identify specifics related to the self-management intervention. This entails defining how the learner will self-manage (e.g., using a paper form, electronic form), how frequently the learner will complete tasks associated with self-management (e.g., every hour, during a particular time of day), and where self-management will take place. Further, it is critical that practitioners identify what types of prompts or cues may be provided to signal engagement in self-management. In some cases, a learner may be provided with a verbal or tactile prompt, with the delivery of the prompt dependent upon learner needs and contextual variables (Koegel et al., 1995).

Next, the practitioner should meet with the learner and describe the self-management intervention. This should involve reviewing definitions of the target behavior and benefits of using the behavior, intervention goals, and intervention specifics. Learners should be provided with materials for self-monitoring skill use, whether these are physical or digital. Materials for self-monitoring should be tailored to individual student needs and contextual variables. Following introduction of intervention materials, learners should engage in discrimination training while self-monitoring. Within discrimination training, learners may first observe others (e.g., practitioner, peers) demonstrating examples and non-examples of the target skill. While observing models, the learner should practice using the self-management materials and feedback should be provided regarding skill accuracy. Learners should then be provided with the opportunity to practice the target skill and use the self-management intervention for their own behavior. Training may be continued until learners demonstrate sufficient accuracy in implementing the intervention.

Following, the self-management intervention should be implemented as developed. During implementation of the intervention, it is critical that practitioners evaluate intervention fidelity and conduct retraining in intervention procedures as needed. Next, regular evaluation of performance should be conducted. Some learners may be able to engage in independent self-evaluation as described earlier in this chapter, whereas other learners may need additional support in determining whether behavioral goals were met. Relatedly, reinforcement should be provided contingent upon meeting behavioral goals. This may be accomplished independently by the learner (i.e., self-reinforcement) or with the support of the practitioner, depending on the needs of the learner.

Final steps to implementation of self-management should include planning for generalization beyond initial implementation settings. If intervention is initially implemented in a home setting, plans should be made to encourage use in school and community settings—ensuring that support and reinforcement for skill use is contacted across all settings. Once the intervention effect is established, practitioners should gradually fade self-management procedures. This may be accomplished by reducing the frequency or intensity of cues for self-management, reducing the frequency of reinforcement, or increasing response requirements. Self-management procedures should continue to be faded until the learner demonstrates skill use independently and consistently over time.

Practical Case Example

LaBroth is a 10-year-old client who has reported difficulty requesting help from his teachers in school when he has trouble completing academic assignments independently in class. Instead, LaBroth is likely to sit quietly at his desk for the entire independent work period and as a result is not making sufficient academic progress. Through consultation with LaBroth's parents and classroom teacher, you develop a self-management intervention package that will enable LaBroth to increase the amount of independent work he is completing with assistance from his teacher. The self-management package includes components of self-monitoring, self-evaluation, and self-reinforcement.

Each day, at the beginning of the 30 min independent math work period, LaBroth will be provided with a MotivAider which has been programmed to vibrate at 3 min intervals. He will also have a small slip of paper with ten empty boxes on it, each one representing one of the 3 min intervals that comprise the 30 min work period. Each time the MotivAider buzzes, LaBroth will determine whether he has been making adequate progress toward task completion or not. If he determines that he has and that he does not require assistance from his teacher, he will put a check in the corresponding box on the slip of paper. If he determines that he is not and that he does require assistance from his teacher he will raise his hand until help is provided. LaBroth's teacher has also agreed to provide him with assistance in a timely manner (i.e., before the next 3 min interval is expired). Once assistance has been provided and LaBroth is once again working independently, his teacher will mark a check in the appropriate interval. Finally, if the timer goes off twice in a row (i.e., two intervals) and LaBroth has not made adequate progress nor asked for assistance from his teacher he will mark those boxes and all consecutive boxes with an X until he either engages the task or requests help. Finally, at the end of the 30-min period, LaBroth will count the number of checks made by himself, his teacher, and any Xs. These data can be used to evaluate the extent to which LaBroth is working independently (his checks), he is working with requests for teacher support (teacher checks), or not working independently or with teacher support (Xs).

Also, to enable a self-reinforcement component, LaBroth is able to earn a small reward from a prize box at home as long as his daily self-management form indicates that he had more checks than Xs. In the future, as LaBroth has success with this system, the number of checks required for reinforcement may be increased. Additionally, although the goal was to at first promote requesting help from his teacher, the goal could also be shifted in the future to require a certain number of independent work checks rather than teacher checks to encourage independent academic work.

Conclusion

Self-management is a performance-based strategy used to increase the frequency and duration of appropriate social behavior in individuals with ASD. It is comprised of three distinct processes, self-monitoring, self-evaluation, and self-reinforcement which together promote generalization of treatment effects across people and settings. Although it may not be appropriate for very young learners (i.e., those younger than school age), it has been identified as an evidence-based practice across a number of systematic reviews and meta-analyses. When combined with acquisition-based teaching strategies (e.g., BST), self-management becomes a powerful strategy to drive learner responding across contexts.

References

Apple, A. L., Billingsley, F., Schwartz, I. S., & Carr, E. G. (2005). Effects of video modeling alone and with self-management on compliment-giving behaviors of children with high-functioning ASD. *Journal of Positive Behavior Interventions, 7*, 33–46.

Carr, M. E., Moore, D. W., & Anderson, A. (2014). Self-management interventions on students with autism: A meta-analysis of single-subject research. *Exceptional Children, 81*, 28–44.

Cooper, J. O., Heron, T. E., & Heward, W. L. (2020). *Applied behavior analysis* (3rd ed.). Pearson.

Davis, J. L., Mason, B. A., Davis, H. S., Mason, R. A., & Crutchfield, S. A. (2016). Self-monitoring interventions for students with ASD: A meta-analysis of school-based research. *Review Journal of Autism and Developmental Disorders, 3*, 196–208.

Eisenberg, N., Spinrad, T. L., & Eggum, N. D. (2010). Emotion-related self-regulation and its relation to children's maladjustment. *Annual Review of Clinical Psychology, 6*, 495–525.

Galbicka, G. (1994). Shaping in the 21st century: Moving percentile schedules into applied settings. *Journal of Applied Behavior Analysis, 27*, 739–760.

Hepburn, S. L., & Wolff, B. C. (2013). Self-regulation in persons with autism spectrum disorders. In K. C. Barrett, N. A. Fox, G. A. Morgan, D. J. Fidler, & L. A. Daunhauer (Eds.), *Handbook of self-regulatory processes in development: New directions and international perspectives* (pp. 429–452). Psychology Press.

Hood, S. A., Olsen, A. E., Luczynski, K. C., & Randle, F. A. (2020). Improving accepting and giving compliments with individuals with developmental disabilities. *Journal of Applied Behavior Analysis, 53*, 1013–1028.

Inzlicht, M., Werner, K. M., Briskin, J. L., & Roberts, B. W. (2021). Integrating models of self-regulation. *Annual Review of Psychology, 72*, 319–345.

Kanfer, F. H. (1977). The many faces of self-control, or behavior modification changes its focus. In R. B. Stuart (Ed.), *Behavioral self-management: Strategies, techniques, and outcomes* (pp. 1–48). Brunner/Mazel.

Koegel, L. K., Koegel, R. L., Hurley, C., & Frea, W. D. (1992). Improving social skills and disruptive behavior in children with autism through self-management. *Journal of Applied Behavior Analysis, 25*, 341–353.

Koegel, R. L., Koegel, L. K., & Parks, D. R. (1995). "Teach the individual" model of generalization: Autonomy through self-management. In R. L. Koegel & L. K. Koegel (Eds.), *Teaching children with autism: Strategies for initiating positive interactions and improving learning opportunities* (pp. 67–77). Brookes.

Lee, S. H., Simpson, R. L., & Shogren, K. A. (2007). Effects and implications of self-management for students with autism: A meta-analysis. *Focus on Autism and Other Developmental Disabilities, 22*, 2–13.
Liu, Y., Moore, D. W., & Anderson, A. (2015). Improving social skills in a child with autism spectrum disorder through self-management training. *Behaviour Change, 32*, 273–284.
McKown, C., Gumbiner, L. M., Russo, N. M., & Lipton, M. (2009). Social-emotional learning skill, self-regulation, and social competence in typically developing and clinic-referred children. *Journal of Clinical Child & Adolescent Psychology, 38*, 858–871.
MotivAider. (2017). *MotivAider®: Making people better, one habit at a time*. (Behavioral Dynamics). Retrieved June 25, 2021, from Habitchange.com: http://habitchange.com/
National Autism Center. (2015). *Findings and conclusions: National standards project, Phase 2*. Retrieved from http://www.nationalautismcenter.org/
Nelson, R. O., & Hayes, S. C. (1981). Theoretical explanations for reactivity in self-monitoring. *Behavior Modification, 5*, 3–14.
Parker, D., & Kamps, D. (2011). Effects of task analysis and self-monitoring for children with autism in multiple social settings. *Focus on Autism and Other Developmental Disabilities, 26*, 131–142.
Peterson, L. D., Young, K. R., West, R. P., & Peterson, M. H. (1999). Effects of student self-management on generalization of student performance to regular classrooms. *Education and Treatment of Children, 22*, 357–372.
Rachlin, H. (1974). Self-control. *Behaviorism, 2*, 94–107.
Radley, K. C., Dart, E. H., Brennan, K. J., Helbig, K. A., Lehman, E. L., Silberman, M., & Mendanhall, K. (2020). Social skills teaching for individuals with autism spectrum disorder: A systematic review. *Advances in Neurodevelopmental Disorders, 4*, 215–226.
Reinecke, D., Newman, B., & Meinberg, D. (1999). Self-management of sharing in three preschoolers with autism. *Education and Training in Mental Retardation and Developmental Disabilities, 34*, 312–317.
Shapiro, E. S., McGonigle, J. J., & Ollendick, T. H. (1980). An analysis of self-assessment and self-reinforcement in a self-managed token economy with mentally retarded children. *Applied Research in Mental Retardation, 1*, 227–240.
Smith, R. L., Eklund, K., & Kilgus, S. P. (2018). Concurrent validity and sensitivity to change of Direct Behavior Rating Single-Item Scales (DBR-SIS) within an elementary sample. *School Psychology Quarterly, 33*, 83.
Stokes, T. F., & Osnes, P. G. (1989). An operant pursuit of generalization. *Behavior Therapy, 20*, 337–355.
Watkins, L., Ledbetter-Cho, K., O'Reilly, M., Barnard-Brak, L., & Garcia-Grau, P. (2019). Interventions for students with autism in inclusive settings: A best-evidence synthesis and meta-analysis. *Psychological Bulletin, 145*, 490.
Zegiob, L., Klukas, N., & Junginger, J. (1978). Reactivity of self-monitoring procedures with retarded adolescents. *American Journal of Mental Deficiency, 83*, 156–163.

Chapter 10
Discrete Trial Teaching

Discrete trial teaching, also called discrete trial training (DTT; e.g., Tarbox & Najdowski, 2008), is a behavior analytic method of instruction first used to teach verbal behavior to children with ASD (Lovaas, 1977; Lovaas & Smith, 1989). Due to its effectiveness in this capacity, DTT has since been used to teach a wider variety of functional, academic, and adaptive behaviors including communication skills (e.g., Koegel et al., 1988), academic responses (e.g., Carroll et al., 2016), and daily living skills (e.g., Downs et al., 2007). Like many of the other strategies discussed in this text, DTT is rooted in Thorndike's Law of Effect (Thorndike, 1927), Skinner's operant conditioning (Skinner, 1963), and applied behavior analysis (e.g., Cooper et al., 2020). Operant conditioning occurs when our voluntary behaviors are shaped by the consequences that follow them, making them more or less likely to be exhibited again in the future. Specifically, those behaviors followed by pleasurable consequences are more likely to occur in the future and those behaviors followed by negative consequences are less likely to occur in the future.

This type of conditioning can occur naturally as clients interact with their environment (e.g., they may be less likely to pet a dog after reaching for one and being bitten); however, DTT takes a more intentional approach to operant conditioning by structuring opportunities for targeted behaviors to contact a pleasurable consequence (i.e., reinforcement), thereby increasing the future likelihood of their occurrence. Furthermore, the opportunities for reinforcement within a DTT paradigm occur at a much more rapid and measured pace than the natural environment would provide, increasing the number of opportunities a client has to respond (e.g., Haydon et al., 2012).

In DTT, each opportunity for the client to exhibit the target behavior is known as a trial, hence the name discrete trial teaching. These trials are the smallest unit of teaching within the instructional paradigm and a single DTT session may see clients responding over many, many trials. For this reason, DTT has sometimes been called "massed-trial instruction" (e.g., Francisco & Hanley, 2012; Majdalany et al., 2014).

K. C Radley, E. H. Dart, *Social Skills Teaching for Individuals with Autism*, Springer Series on Child and Family Studies,
https://doi.org/10.1007/978-3-030-91665-7_10

This practice is supported by research demonstrating that a higher number of opportunities to respond is linked to increased academic engagement and client outcomes (e.g., Common et al., 2020). Fast-paced instruction through brief intertrial intervals are one of the core components of effective DTT. The rest of this chapter will break down the other critical elements of DTT in great detail, providing readers with a thorough understanding of the behavior analytic components and therapeutic mechanisms of DTT. We will also provide a review of the literature supporting DTT to promote social skill acquisition in individuals with ASD, one of its most popular applications. Finally, we will conclude with a practical case example and chapter summary.

Critical Elements of DTT

As mentioned previously, DTT is rooted in principles of operant conditioning and applied behavior analysis. Specifically, every trial within DTT is composed of the same three elements: (1) an antecedent prompt signaling to the learner that a specific response is requested; (2) the response exhibited by the learner; and (3) reinforcement contingent upon the response. These three components make up the three-term contingency (e.g., Albers & Greer, 1991) underlying operant conditioning and make up the fundamental therapeutic mechanism supporting DTT. Recall that responses contacting reinforcement are more likely to be exhibited again in the future. Next, we will describe these three components in greater detail.

Discriminative Stimulus

A discriminative stimulus is any stimulus that signals to an individual that a specific behavior is likely to contact reinforcement (Cooper et al., 2020). Discriminative stimuli are often abbreviated as S^D (pronounced "ess-dee") and form the first part of the three-term contingency referenced earlier. One example of an S^D from a naturalistic contingency includes door signage indicating that a bathroom is just through the door. This stimulus signals to us that our bathroom-seeking behavior will be reinforced for proceeding through the door. Another example is the question posed by a teacher to students: "Who can tell me the name of the line opposite the right angle in a right triangle?" signaling that the response of "hypotenuse" will likely contact reinforcement. Keep in mind that S^Ds are not perfect indicators that reinforcement is available. For example, the door with the bathroom signage may be locked, preventing entry and the student raising their hand to answer the teacher's question may not be called upon. Instead, S^Ds simply signal to us that a particular response is likely to be reinforced when they are present and likely not to be reinforced when they are not (e.g., you may wander through an unmarked door in your search for a bathroom and find one).

It is also important to note that stimuli do not function universally as S^Ds for all individuals. It is through our unique learning histories that previously neutral stimuli come to take on discriminative properties; however, individuals learning in similar environments (e.g., home, community, culture) are likely to learn many of the same contingencies and the S^Ds that signal their availability (e.g., bathroom signage). When it comes to teaching social behavior within a DTT paradigm, it is necessary to consider the relevant S^Ds that signal to us which social response is likely to be reinforced. The goal of DTT is to create new three-term contingencies that are likely to generalize to settings outside of the teaching setting. This is accomplished by repeatedly pairing the relevant S^D with the appropriate response and reinforcement. In the end, the goal is to shape a neutral stimulus into an S^D that signals to the learner that a particular social behavior will contact reinforcement. Furthermore, because DTT is fundamentally an acquisition intervention (i.e., targeting skill acquisition rather than performance), it is critical that the S^Ds chosen during the teaching process are likely to be encountered by learners once they leave the instructional setting. For example, consider the social skill of identifying oneself by name. This is an important early step in forming new relationships with others. If you wanted to teach a learner to exhibit this behavior using DTT, it would not be appropriate to select "Say your name" as an S^D. Although we may encounter the S^D "Say your name" in naturalistic environments and it may be reinforcing to respond to this S^D with our own names it is likely not going to generalize to many social situations. Instead, it might be more appropriate to select the S^D "Who are you?" or "What is your name?" as these are more likely to appear as S^Ds in naturalistic settings when individuals meet each other for the first time.

There is some debate about whether to use a range of antecedent prompts (e.g., "What's your name?" and "Who are you?") or one prompt when teaching a skill using DTT. The single prompt proponents suggest that too much variability in the form of antecedent prompts may prohibit learning by slowing the establishment of clear three-term contingencies (e.g., Grow & LeBlanc, 2013). Others suggest that while variability in prompt form may impede initial acquisition, it is critical if learners are expected to exhibit the skills learned in DTT across the wide variety of settings and naturalistic stimuli they are likely to encounter once instruction concludes (Leaf et al., 2016). The most practical recommendation is to begin instruction of a new skill with a single prompt and allow the learner to demonstrate mastery with that prompt before introducing variability by using multiple exemplars (Stokes & Baer, 1977).

Response

As mentioned previously, DTT is primarily used to promote skill acquisition rather than to increase performance of an acquired skill. Because of this, the appropriate responses to the targeted S^Ds are not likely to be within a learner's behavioral repertoire. In other words, the first time a learner is presented with the S^D of "What is your name?" they may not respond at all or they may respond incorrectly because they do not know what constitutes an appropriate response. Thus, teachers using DTT may find themselves endlessly repeating a S^D waiting for the learner to exhibit a correct response or any response at all. To address this issue, it is most common for instructors using DTT to use a hierarchy of response prompts, with the initial S^D (e.g., "What is your name?") being just the first of several prompts.

Prompting hierarchies structure a progression of additional prompts that are subsequently exhibited by the DTT instructor if the learner does not exhibit an appropriate response to the initial S^D and the subsequent prompts. There are several different types of prompts that can be given (i.e., verbal, gestural, model, and physical) and they are categorized based on their topography. Verbal prompts are often used as initial S^Ds, particularly when teaching social skills as these are the most commonly occurring type of naturalistic social cue. Verbal prompts may also be used to supplement the initial S^D in the absence of an appropriate response. For example, if a learner named Keith fails to exhibit an appropriate response to the S^D "What is your name?", the teacher may repeat the S^D followed immediately by an additional verbal prompt (i.e., "What is your name? K-"). The addition of the k sound prompts the learner to exhibit the correct response (i.e., "Keith"). Verbal prompts can be taken to the level of providing the entire correct response (i.e., "What is your name? Keith") should that level of prompting be necessary for a learner.

Gestural prompts include any physical gesture made by the teacher to signal to the learner what the appropriate response may entail. Examples of gestural prompts include pointing, facial orientation, and head shaking or nodding. Consider the statement "Look at this" as a possible S^D for recruiting joint attention. Pointing at the object of interest is an example of a gestural prompt that could follow the S^D. Model prompts involve the teacher demonstrating the appropriate behavior for the learner. For example, given the S^D "Touch your head." a subsequent model prompt would have the teacher touching their own head to demonstrate to the learner what the appropriate response looks like. Lastly, physical prompts require the teacher to use hand-over-hand guidance to facilitate appropriate responding by the learner. Using the S^D "Touch your head" again as an example, a physical prompt would have the teacher take the learner's hand and gently touch it to the learner's own head, physically simulating the appropriate response.

Within a DTT paradigm, response prompts are typically arranged in a hierarchy by their level of intrusiveness to the learner. Common hierarchies include most-to-least prompting and least-to-most prompting, describing the starting point and direction in which the prompts change by their level of intrusiveness. For example, a least-to-most hierarchy might start first with the verbal S^D (e.g., "Look at that!") followed by a gestural prompt (e.g., pointing toward object of interest), model prompt (e.g., teacher making exaggerated head turn toward and eye contact with object of interest), and physical (e.g., teacher turning learner's head toward object of interest). On the other hand, a most-to-least prompt would reverse the order with the exception of the S^D, which always comes first and is almost always repeated prior to each new prompt given. Learners who do not respond correctly to the initial S^D are given the S^D again paired with the next prompt in the hierarchy. Prompting continues in this way until the learner exhibits a correct response or the teacher has exhausted the most intensive prompt (i.e., full physical prompt). It is common to note the level of prompting needed for each trial to determine whether learners are becoming dependent on certain types of prompts and whether progress is trending toward independent responding (i.e., requiring no additional prompts other than the S^D).

Research investigating the relative effectiveness of the different prompt types and prompting hierarchies within DTT suggest that differences are likely idiosyncratic (e.g., Seaver & Bourret, 2014). For all prompt types, it is very common for the initial antecedent prompt to be repeated with whichever prompt is being used. In this way, the initial antecedent prompt is still paired with the correct response and subsequent reinforcement. Additionally, instructors can build a fixed or progressive time delay into their prompting procedures, meaning learners are given a brief period of time (e.g., 3 s) to exhibit the correct response before a subsequent prompt is provided. This time period is meant to reduce learner dependence on prompts and allow them to contact reinforcement more quickly should they exhibit the response independently compared to waiting for the next prompt (e.g., Soulaga et al., 2008).

Consequence

The last component to consider within the DTT paradigm is the consequence following a learner's correct response. Within a trial, when a learner exhibits a correct response it should be reinforced in order to strengthen the three-term contingency (i.e., S^D, response, reinforcement). In other words, it is the reinforcing consequence that signals to the learner that their response was appropriate and is likely to produce additional reinforcement in the future, sustaining their behavior. When skills are first taught in a DTT program it is very common to use a thick schedule of reinforcement (e.g., FR1 or continuous reinforcement). In an FR1 schedule, every appropriate response by the learner is reinforced. This is not sustainable over a long period of time and certainly not reflective of naturalistic settings (recall the example of attempting to enter a bathroom and finding the door locked); however, it is likely to drive rapid skill acquisition. Once the learner reliably exhibits the appropriate response when the teacher presents the S^D, the schedule of reinforcement can be thinned (e.g., FR3, FR10) or switched to a schedule that more closely resembles naturalistic settings (e.g., VR3). The stimuli used to reinforce responding can vary and depend on what is accessible and appropriate for a particular learner.

It is common for teachers using DTT to condition their own presence and social attention as a reinforcing stimulus. This process is known as pairing and it is a way for teachers to provide reinforcement to learners without relying on excessive delivery of edible stimuli (e.g., candy) or tangible stimuli (e.g., iPad access). Lugo et al. (2017) describe a systematic process that includes close physical proximity, frequent verbal praise, reflections of the learner's verbalizations, imitation of the learner, description of the learner's play behavior, and initiation and creation of play with the learner. Additionally, preference assessments and reinforcer assessments (e.g., Cannella et al., 2005) can provide insight into what stimuli may be used within a DTT program to reinforce correct responding. Finally, token economies (Matson & Boisjoli, 2009), in which arbitrary stimuli (i.e., tokens) acquire reinforcing properties because they can be exchanged for primary reinforcers (i.e., edible or tangible stimuli), have been used frequently to establish and maintain DTT programs (Haq et al., 2015).

Empirical Support

Interventions based in DTT have generally been found to be effective for promoting skill acquisition in children with ASD. In summarizing research in DTT, several meta-analyses have reported positive outcomes for individuals with ASD who are exposed to DTT interventions. In one example, Kane et al. (2010) evaluated the effectiveness of spoken language interventions developed for children with ASD. A total of 22 studies were included in the study, which included interventions that consisted of either contrived (i.e., DTT) or naturalistic opportunities to learn and practice skills. Overall, the meta-analysis found that both contrived and naturalistic approaches resulted in skill acquisition and use in both training and generalization settings. However, DTT-based approaches resulted in greater skill generalization for children with ASD—highlighting the utility of this approach for promoting skill use.

In another meta-analysis, Virués-Ortega (2010) examined the effectiveness of long-term, comprehensive ABA interventions in children with diagnoses of ASD or pervasive developmental disability—not otherwise specified. A total of 22 studies focusing on DTT-based intervention were included in the meta-analysis. Overall, the researchers found medium to large positive treatment effects for DTT interventions for "intellectual functioning, language development, acquisition of daily living skills and social functioning in children with autism" (Virués-Ortega, 2010, p. 387). Similarly, Peters-Scheffer et al. (2011) evaluated the effectiveness of Early Intensive Behavioral Intervention (EIBI), which included DTT, in children with ASD. In the 11 included studies, experimental groups that received EIBI "outperformed the control groups on IQ, non-verbal IQ, expressive and receptive language, and adaptive behavior" (Peters-Scheffer et al., 2011, p. 60). Taken together, these meta-analyses provide strong support for the overall effectiveness of DTT in promoting a range of positive outcomes for individuals with ASD. Given the strength of research supporting DTT and related intervention strategies, the National Autism Center's (2015) National Standards Project identified Behavioral Interventions, which included DTT, and Comprehensive Behavioral Treatments, of which DTT is often a component, as evidence-based practices for individuals with ASD.

Although some meta-analyses have noted positive outcomes for social functioning, no meta-analyses have exclusively summarized research evaluating DTT for promoting social outcomes. Despite this, numerous individual studies provide insight into the utility of DTT as a social skills teaching strategy. For example, Francisco and Hanley (2012) evaluated the effect of social skills teaching via DTT for two preschool-age children with ASD. A total of three different social skills were addressed as part of training. To set up trials, the researchers would arrange the environment in such a way to allow for an opportunity to demonstrate the target skill. If an incorrect response was demonstrated, the researcher would provide error correction—consisting of describing and modeling the target social skill. Following, the researcher would provide an additional opportunity to demonstrate the skill. Correct demonstrations of the skill resulted in descriptive praise, whereas further incorrect demonstrations resulted in reteaching as previously described. Results of the study found that, when trials were separated by relatively long intertrial intervals, acquisition of social responses was slow. However, when intertrial intervals were initially short, acquisition of skills was found to be more rapid.

In another example, Koegel et al. (2009) investigated the delivery of reinforcers with embedded social interactions within a trial-based framework. As part of the intervention, an adult would present a potential reinforcer as a means of engaging a participant with ASD during 10-min probe sessions. Reinforcers with embedded social interaction were defined as the adult engaging in the requested reinforcer with the participant. For example, if the participant requested "jump" after being shown a trampoline, the adult would jump on the trampoline with the participant. Results of the study indicated greater self-initiated social engagement when reinforcers had embedded social interactions, with lower levels of engagement being observed when reinforcers were not embedded. Similar results were observed with respect to nonverbal dyadic orienting of participants when presented with reinforcers with embedded social interactions.

Shabani et al. (2002) investigated the use of tactile prompting as a means of increasing social initiations in children with ASD, with initial training provided using a DTT format. In the study, three children with ASD engaged in training sessions in which a tactile prompting device cued the use of a social interaction statement at 1 min intervals. During this time, a researcher sat across from a participant and, when the tactile prompt was activated, provided a verbal model of an initiation statement. If the participant initiated the model, they were provided with an edible item. This process was repeated, with the verbal models of the participant being faded until the participant independently demonstrated the initiation statement when the tactile prompt was activated. Following training, the tactile device continued to be used during 10-min free-play sessions. Compared to baseline sessions, intervention session data reveal a substantially greater number of both verbal initiations and responses for all participants, suggesting that the intervention was effective in promoting social engagement of participants.

DTT has also been utilized in conjunction with technology within social skills teaching interventions. Yun et al. (2017) designed a robot system that assisted a clinician in DTT to promote emotion recognition and use of eye contact. Each intervention session was 30–40 min in duration and consisted of delivery of multiple trials for target skill use. During a trial, the robot would provide social reinforcement to participants upon correct responses (e.g., "I'm pleased that you can recognize my feelings"). Incorrect responses resulted in the robot offering the participant encouragement. Results of the study indicated that the duration of eye contact and the number of emotions correctly identified increased. Additionally, parent reported play behaviors were noted to improve while reports of general behavioral and emotional symptoms decreased. Overall, the results indicate that this modality of DTT was effective in promoting social outcomes for children with ASD.

Practical Case Example

Eduardo is a 5-year-old male with a diagnosis with ASD. He receives school-based support for social skills, but also attends an early intervention program at a community-based clinic after school. At the present time, Eduardo's primary intervention goal is increasing the demonstration of appropriate social interactions. Eduardo often attempts to initiate interactions with peers and adults, but the topography of initiation often results in unsuccessful bids for attention. More specifically, Eduardo will often hit or inappropriately touch conversation partners as a means of gaining attention—resulting in peer avoidance or ignoring of initiation attempts.

Through consultation with Eduardo's parents it was determined that he will receive 1 h of DTT each day after school to focus on the acquisition of initiating appropriate social responses. Each day, Eduardo attends a DTT session delivered by a behavior analyst in a clinical setting. The sessions begin with a 5-min warm-up period whereby the behavior analyst and Eduardo play with a variety of toys and other tangible stimuli available in the room. Once the warm-up period ends, Eduardo is asked to sit at a small table in the room. The behavior analyst also sits in a chair across from Eduardo at the same table. Together, they spend the next 5 min discussing how to appropriately ask others to talk with you (i.e., getting their attention and saying "Let's talk!"; not hitting them). Because the focus of these sessions is on Eduardo's appropriate social initiation, the S^D for requesting social interaction involves the behavior analyst engaging in an activity without Eduardo (e.g., paperwork, manipulating some toy or other object) as this most closely resembles the situations in which Eduardo is likely to attempt to recruit social attention in more naturalistic settings. Any inappropriate response by Eduardo (i.e., hitting to gain attention) is ignored during these sessions.

Once the behavior analyst begins engaging in the activity, the first trial begins. If after 10 s Eduardo does not exhibit an appropriate social initiation (e.g., "Let's talk!"), the behavior analyst turns to Eduardo and then points to himself to signal that he is available for social interaction. If Eduardo exhibits an appropriate social initiation, the behavior analyst provides verbal praise and the two engage in conversation for 2 min. If not, the behavior analyst moves on to the next most intrusive prompt (i.e., tapping Eduardo on the shoulder and then pointing to himself). This process continues until: (1) Eduardo initiates social interaction or (2) the behavior analyst provides the most intrusive prompt (i.e., a verbal prompt of "Eduardo say 'Let's talk!'"). Regardless of the level of prompt necessary, any appropriate response by Eduardo is met with social praise from the behavior analyst and 2 min of conversation. Once the 2 min conversational period is over, a new trial begins once the behavior analyst returns to the activity without Eduardo by saying "Ok, I have to get back to this now." Over the course of the hour, the behavior analyst is able to conduct 20 trials in this way in addition to the warm-up period, brief didactic instruction, and a short break at the halfway point of the hour.

Once Eduardo is able to repeatedly demonstrate appropriate bids for initiation in the treatment setting, the behavior analyst decides to evaluate whether the newly acquired skill will generalize to novel conversation partners and settings. In order to do so, the behavior analyst invites Eduardo's father to present the same cue for social engagement. During the first trial, Eduardo hits his father in order to recruit his attention. Upon doing so, reteaching is presented in a manner identical to initial instruction with the behavior analyst. Next, Eduardo's father is encouraged to present the cue for social engagement. Instead of hitting, Eduardo states "Let's talk!," to which Eduardo's father responds by engaging in conversation. Cues for engagement are presented by Eduardo's father multiple times across multiple sessions, with Eduardo demonstrating appropriate bids for attention on all subsequent trials. The therapist then works with Eduardo and his father to identify times at which Eduardo may practice the skill outside of the clinic. Together, they identify times at school, home, and in the community in which Eduardo may initiate interactions with peers or adults. Eduardo's father is encouraged to observe skill use when possible and provide feedback regarding skill use. Over several weeks, Eduardo is observed by his father to improve initiations in generalized settings. Eduardo, his father, and the behavior analyst decide that intervention may now target other skills.

Conclusion

In conclusion, DTT is an evidence-based instructional paradigm that has been used to teach a wide variety of skills to learners of all different abilities; however, it is very commonly used as a skill acquisition intervention to teach social behavior to individuals with ASD. By intentionally arranging three-term contingencies, providing support through the use of prompts, and providing learners many opportunities to respond, DTT can be used to promote rapid acquisition of social skills. The empirical basis supporting DTT for this purpose indicates that it is generally effective, particularly for foundational social skills such as social initiation, eye contact, and duration of social engagement. Learners who do not already possess or exhibit these foundational skills may benefit the most from the structure and intensity of a DTT program.

References

Albers, A. E., & Greer, R. D. (1991). Is the three-term contingency trial a predictor of effective instruction? *Journal of Behavioral Education, 1*, 337–354.

Cannella, H. I., O'Reilly, M. F., & Lancioni, G. E. (2005). Choice and preference assessment research with people with severe to profound developmental disabilities: A review of the literature. *Research in Developmental Disabilities, 26*, 1–15.

Carroll, R. A., Kodak, T., & Adolf, K. J. (2016). Effect of delayed reinforcement on skill acquisition during discrete-trial instruction: Implications for treatment-integrity errors in academic settings. *Journal of Applied Behavior Analysis, 49*, 176–181.
Common, E. A., Lane, K. L., Cantwell, E. D., Brunsting, N. C., Oakes, W. P., Germer, K. A., & Bross, L. A. (2020). Teacher-delivered strategies to increase students' opportunities to respond: A systematic methodological review. *Behavioral Disorders, 45*, 67–84.
Cooper, J. O., Heron, T. E., & Heward, W. L. (2020). *Applied behavior analysis* (3rd ed.). Pearson.
Downs, A., Robyn, C. D., Johansen, M., & Fossum, M. (2007). Using discrete trial teaching within a public preschool program to facilitate skill development in students with developmental disabilities. *Education & Treatment of Children, 30*, 1–27.
Francisco, M. T., & Hanley, G. P. (2012). An evaluation of progressively increasing intertrial intervals on the acquisition and generalization of three social skills. *Journal of Applied Behavior Analysis, 45*, 137–142.
Grow, L., & LeBlanc, L. (2013). Teaching receptive language skills. *Behavior Analysis in Practice, 6*, 56–75.
Haq, S. S., Kodak, T., Kurtz-Nelson, E., Porritt, M., Rush, K., & Cariveau, T. (2015). Comparing the effects of massed and distributed practice on skill acquisition for children with autism. *Journal of Applied Behavior Analysis, 48*, 454–459.
Haydon, T., Macsuga-Gage, A. S., Simonsen, B., & Hawkins, R. (2012). Opportunities to respond: A key component of effective instruction. *Beyond Behavior, 22*, 23–31.
Kane, M., Connell, J. E., & Pellecchia, M. (2010). A quantitative analysis of language interventions for children with autism. *The Behavior Analyst Today, 11*, 128.
Koegel, R. L., O'Dell, M., & Dunlap, G. (1988). Producing speech use in nonverbal autistic children by reinforcing attempts. *Journal of Autism and Developmental Disorders, 18*, 525–538.
Koegel, R. L., Vernon, T. W., & Koegel, L. K. (2009). Improving social initiations in young children with autism using reinforcers with embedded social interactions. *Journal of Autism and Developmental Disorders, 39*, 1240–1251.
Leaf, J. B., Cihon, J. H., Leaf, R., McEachin, J., & Taubman, M. (2016). A progressive approach to discrete trial teaching: Some current guidelines. *International Electronic Journal of Elementary Education, 9*, 361–372.
Lovaas, O. I. (1977). *The autistic child: Language development through behavior modification*. Irvington.
Lovaas, O. I., & Smith, T. (1989). A comprehensive behavioral theory of autistic children: Paradigm for research and treatment. *Journal of Behavior Therapy and Experimental Psychiatry, 20*, 17–29.
Lugo, A. M., King, M. L., Lamphere, J. C., & McArdle, P. E. (2017). Developing procedures to improve therapist–child rapport in early intervention. *Behavior Analysis in Practice, 10*, 395–401.
Majdalany, L. M., Wilder, D. A., Greif, A., Mathisen, D., & Saini, V. (2014). Comparing massed-trial instruction, distributed-trial instruction, and task interspersal to teach tacts to children with autism spectrum disorders. *Journal of Applied Behavior Analysis, 47*, 657–662.
Matson, J. L., & Boisjoli, J. A. (2009). The token economy for children with intellectual disability and/or autism: A review. *Research in Developmental Disabilities, 30*, 240–248.
National Autism Center. (2015). *Findings and conclusions: National standards project, Phase 2*. Retrieved from http://www.nationalautismcenter.org/
Peters-Scheffer, N., Didden, R., Korzilius, H., & Sturmey, P. (2011). A meta-analytic study on the effectiveness of comprehensive ABA-based early intervention programs for children with autism spectrum disorders. *Research in Autism Spectrum Disorders, 5*, 60–69.
Seaver, J. L., & Bourret, J. C. (2014). An evaluation of response prompts for teaching behavior chains. *Journal of Applied Behavior Analysis, 47*, 777–792.
Shabani, D. B., Katz, R. C., Wilder, D. A., Beauchamp, K., Taylor, C. R., & Fischer, K. J. (2002). Increasing social initiations in children with autism: Effects of a tactile prompt. *Journal of Applied Behavior Analysis, 35*, 79–83.

Skinner, B. F. (1963). Operant behavior. *American Psychologist, 18*, 503.

Soulaga, D., Leaf, J. B., Taubman, M., McEachin, J., & Leaf, R. B. (2008). A comparison of flexible prompt fading and constant time delay for five children with autism. *Research in Autism Spectrum Disorders, 2*, 753–765.

Stokes, T. F., & Baer, D. M. (1977). An implicit technology of generalization. *Journal of Applied Behavior Analysis, 10*, 349–367.

Tarbox, R. S., & Najdowski, A. C. (2008). Discrete trial training as a teaching paradigm. In J. K. Luiselli, D. C. Russo, W. P. Christian, & S. M. Wilcyznski (Eds.), *Effective practices for children with autism: Educational and behavior support interventions that work* (pp. 181–194). Oxford University Press.

Thorndike, E. L. (1927). The law of effect. *The American Journal of Psychology, 39*, 212–222.

Virués-Ortega, J. (2010). Applied behavior analytic intervention for autism in early childhood: Meta-analysis, meta-regression and dose–response meta-analysis of multiple outcomes. *Clinical Psychology Review, 30*, 387–399.

Yun, S. S., Choi, J., Park, S. K., Bong, G. Y., & Yoo, H. (2017). Social skills training for children with autism spectrum disorder using a robotic behavioral intervention system. *Autism Research, 10*, 1306–1323.

Chapter 11
Other Behavior Analytic Strategies

Behavior analysis is a scientific field concerned with the understanding and application of Skinner's theoretical work on human behavior and operant conditioning (Skinner, 1971). The field is often split into two halves, one concerned with scientific understanding of the basic principles of behavior (i.e., experimental analysis of behavior; Skinner, 1966; Fantino & Logan, 1979) and the other concerned with the application of those principles to improve the human condition (i.e., applied behavior analysis; Baer et al., 1968). Applied behavior analysis (ABA) is conceptually consistent with Skinner's work and the new knowledge generated through the more basic experimental analysis of behavior; however, it emphasizes effective, practical, and generalizable applications of this knowledge rather than the pursuit of fundamental understanding (Baer et al., 1987). Although ABA is broad, covering topics such as environmental protection (e.g., Lehman & Geller, 2004), consumer behavior (e.g., Foxall, 2010), and public health (e.g., Winett et al., 1991), it has notably honed its focus over the last 70 years to the treatment of social and behavioral issues associated with ASD (Axelrod et al., 2012).

The preceding chapters of this text have described individual intervention strategies that are effective in addressing social skills acquisition and performance deficits. Although all of them could be described behavior analytically in terms of their effectiveness, not all were developed intentionally from a behavior analytic framework (e.g., Social Narratives; Chap. 5). This chapter will describe three distinct intervention strategies (i.e., differential reinforcement, chaining, and group contingencies) that were born out of behavior analysis and have been used to address the social behavior of individuals with ASD. Each strategy and their subtypes will be described along with evidence to support their use for this purpose and each will be followed by a brief practical example of their application.

K. C Radley, E. H. Dart, *Social Skills Teaching for Individuals with Autism*, Springer Series on Child and Family Studies,
https://doi.org/10.1007/978-3-030-91665-7_11

Differential Reinforcement

Differential reinforcement is a treatment strategy that combines two distinct components: (1) identification and extinction of a target behavior and (2) identification and reinforcement of a replacement behavior. Operant extinction is the process by which a behavior's source of reinforcement is identified (e.g., peer attention, escape from aversive tasks) and the functional link between the behavior and its reinforcer is severed. In other words, engaging in the behavior no longer produces the reinforcement it did in the past. For example, consider the case of a child who engages in verbally aggressive behavior to get access to a coveted item from a peer. Historically, this child's behavior has always, or nearly always, resulted in them getting access to the item. In this case, the aggressive behavior is functional for the child, allowing them access to items that they want and maintaining its occurrence. Operant extinction would require one or more environmental manipulations to prevent the child's aggressive behavior from getting them access to the coveted item. This may involve immediately returning taken items to peers and instructing peers not to turn over items in the face of the child's verbal aggression. Note that extinction does not necessarily involve blocking or stopping the target behavior, only blocking access to its functional consequence; however, response blocking is commonly combined with differential reinforcement (e.g., Call et al., 2011). The result of extinction is a reduction in the target behavior as the individual learns that it is no longer functional. Thus, differential reinforcement is most applicable when learners may be engaging in inappropriate social behavior.

The second component of differential reinforcement is the identification and reinforcement of the replacement behavior. As the extinction component works to reduce or eliminate the learner's inappropriate or undesirable behavior, the reinforcement component works to increase a different behavior. To maximize the effectiveness of differential reinforcement programs, the reinforcer available to the learner for exhibiting the replacement behavior should be the same as the reinforcer previously contacted by the target behavior. In this way, learners are taught to engage in different behaviors to continue accessing the things that they find reinforcing. Keep in mind that without any additional teaching procedures, differential reinforcement strategies are best suited to address performance deficits as it is often assumed that the replacement behavior is in the learner's repertoire. If this is not the case, consider engaging in behavioral skills training (see Chap. 4) or some other teaching procedure to ensure the learner has acquired the behavior selected as the replacement. The specific behavior that is selected for replacement determines which subtype of differential reinforcement is being implemented.

Differential Reinforcement of Other (DRO) Behavior Under differential reinforcement of other (DRO) behavior, learners contact reinforcement for engaging in any behavior that is not the target behavior. In other words, it is the absence of the target behavior that earns reinforcement and learners are free to engage in any other behavior, there is no specific replacement. Thus, DRO has the effect of reducing a specific target behavior without targeting a corresponding replacement behavior to increase. Typically, learners must refrain from engaging in the target behavior for a specific amount of time (e.g., 1 min interval) before reinforcement is earned and each interval represents another opportunity for reinforcement. Weston and colleagues (2018) conducted a systematic review of the DRO literature aimed at reducing challenging behaviors of individuals with ASD, synthesizing the results of 45 studies on the topic. They found that DRO was implemented commonly by itself or in combination with other differential reinforcement procedures (i.e., DRA), self-monitoring (see Chap. 9), token economies, and response blocking procedures. The DRO intervals were most commonly fixed, meaning they were consistent in length (e.g., 1 min) across the entire treatment session. Surprisingly, only 30% of the studies matched the reinforcement earned under the DRO schedule to the reinforcer identified as maintaining the target behavior, suggesting that a potent enough reinforcer available through a DRO can overcome the reinforcing value of continuing to engage in the target behavior. Overall, they identified DRO as an effective intervention strategy for individuals with ASD (PND = 0.78).

Konczak and Johnson (1983) used DRO to reduce the inappropriate verbalizations (e.g., threats, inappropriate laughter, bizarre noises) of a 42-year-old client in a vocational setting. Under the DRO intervention, the client was able to earn a token and praise from a supervisor every 60 s interval during which they refrained from engaging in inappropriate verbalizations. The client was able to exchange ten tokens for paid overtime, free time, or preferred snacks. The results of the study demonstrate a quick and clear decrease in intervals containing inappropriate verbalizations which were maintained throughout a follow-up phase. Konczak and Johnson note, as recommended by Repp et al. (1975), that the interval selected within a DRO treatment package should be lower than the pre-treatment rate of the target behavior to make sure that the learner is capable of contacting reinforcement. That is, if a learner was exhibiting a target behavior every 30 s, it would not be appropriate to select a DRO interval of 3 min as it is unlikely the learner would be successful.

Differential Reinforcement of Appropriate/Alternative (DRA) Behavior In contrast to DRO, a specific replacement behavior is identified for reinforcement under a DRA procedure. This replacement behavior is often conceptualized as an alternative or appropriate means to access reinforcement previously contacted by the inappropriate target behavior. Think back to the previous example of the child engaging in verbal aggression to access preferred items held by peers. In a DRA arrangement, the replacement behavior might be appropriate requesting (e.g., "May I have a turn with that, please?"), which would then be reinforced with access to the requested item. The learner still contacts the reinforcement sought through the target behavior but are doing so using a behavior that is considered appropriate. MacNaul and Neely (2018) conducted a systematic review of DRA procedures for individuals with ASD and found that the most common alternative behavior targeted was communicative (e.g., picture exchange, vocal response, or a combination of the two) to request access to a preferred reinforcer, suggesting their usefulness in teaching social behaviors. Further, they found that the extinction component of DRA was not always necessary to drive increases in the replacement behavior.

Johnson et al. (2017) investigated the effectiveness of a DRA procedure for three boys diagnosed with ASD who were learning to engage in foundational social behaviors. The target behavior was therapist prompted responses within a discrete trial paradigm and the alternative replacement behavior was unprompted responses within the same paradigm. In other words, the learners were eligible to receive reinforcement when they emitted unprompted responses rather than therapist prompted responses. Also, instead of putting therapist prompted responses on extinction, Johnson et al. (2017) manipulated the quality, magnitude, and schedule of reinforcement across the two response types, making it more reinforcing for participants to exhibit unprompted responses. That is, the higher quality, higher magnitude, or less effortful reinforcement was available for unprompted responses and the lower quality, lower magnitude, and more effortful reinforcement was available for prompted responses. Generally, they found that manipulating reinforcer quality (e.g., highly preferred vs. less preferred) within a DRA arrangement resulted in the quickest and most efficient skill acquisition. These findings are consistent with other studies examining differential reinforcement without a true extinction component (e.g., MacNaul & Neely, 2018).

Differential Reinforcement of Low/High (DRL/H) Rates of Behavior DRL/H Unlike DRO and DRA, the replacement behavior under DRL and DRH is the same as the target behavior with the caveat that it is only occurring under or over a prespecified rate. DRL and DRH are useful when it is desirable for a learner to continue to exhibit a behavior but perhaps at a lower or higher frequency than they currently do. Consider the example of an individual who asks questions of their peers 20 times per minute. Although there is nothing wrong with asking questions, the individual may be doing so at a rate that might prevent meaningful social interaction and a decrease might be desirable. Thus, DRL involves providing learners access to reinforcement so long as the target behavior occurs fewer times than a criterion frequency within a set period of time (e.g., no more than 30 times an hour). Conversely, DRH involves providing learners access to reinforcement so long as the target behavior occurs more times than a criterion frequency within a set period of time (e.g., no less than three times per minute). Alternatively, the reinforcement criterion can be based upon the time passing between responses (e.g., at least 30 s, no more than 30 s) or the frequency within intervals (e.g., no more than three times each minute, no more than three times each minute). The decision to use one over the other depends on the specific learner's needs and the behavior being targeted.

Gadaire et al. (2017) examined the effectiveness of a DRL intervention within a social skills teaching program for five children with ASD. They targeted positive comments and appropriate physical behavior across the five children. All participants were observed to be engaging in excessive levels of these behaviors during social skills lessons, impeding instruction. Participants had to exhibit two or fewer positive comments over a 5-min session or engage in five or fewer instances of appropriate physical contact to receive access to token reinforcement during the social skills lessons. They found that the DRL procedure successfully reduced the children's appropriate behavior below baseline levels to a more manageable level.

These decreases continued through a contingency only phase where they were not given explicit rules about how to behave as well as through a maintenance phase with no contingency in place.

Case Example Duska is a 9-year-old child with a diagnosis of ASD who engages in inappropriate verbal and physical behaviors in an attempt to access snacks from the pantry in her home. Specifically, Duska yells and throws things toward her caregivers until they ask if she would like something to eat and ultimately brings her a snack. Through consultation with Duska and her caregivers it is decided that a DRA contingency will be put into place to address the behavior. Duska is first taught the appropriate behavior selected to replace her current inappropriate behavior. Specifically, Duska's mother tells her that if she wants a snack she can either say "Snack please" or hand her mother one of several cards with a picture of her preferred snacks on them. The two then practice these behaviors to make sure everyone understands how the replacement behaviors will function. In the home, Duska's mother is asked to ignore all yelling and throwing of objects and not engage Duska in conversation related to food when these behaviors occur. Simultaneously, Duska's mother is asked to facilitate her access to food should Duska engage in one of the two appropriate replacement behaviors. Additionally, Duska's mother has decided to layer on a DRL contingency whereby Duska is able to earn a token every hour so long as she does not request more than one snack. These tokens can then be exchanged for small prizes at the end of each day. After implementation of these two differential reinforcement programs, Duska's mother reported that Duska's yelling and throwing objects has decreased, her appropriate snack requesting has increased, and she is requesting snacks at an appropriate rate.

Chaining

As described in Chap. 2, task analysis describes the process of breaking down complex, multistep skills into smaller steps. Chaining is an instructional strategy that relies on task analyses and involves teaching complex skills one step at a time, with skills being taught by themselves within a behavioral sequence. To provide an example, chaining may be used to teach the steps to preparing a pizza. First, a learner may be taught to shape the dough while being supported in all other steps of pizza making. Once the learner is able to complete this step accurately and independently, they would be taught to spread the sauce on the dough—practicing both independent shaping and spreading the sauce and being supported in completing the remaining tasks. Next, the learner may learn to sprinkle shredded cheese on top of the sauce. They would then be provided the opportunity to complete shaping, spreading the sauce, and sprinkling the cheese independently. Finally, the steps for putting on pepperoni would be taught and the entire sequence would be practiced independently. Chaining may be used to teach any complex skill, inclusive of social behaviors. Researchers have generally identified three types of chaining strategies: forward chaining, backward chaining, and total-task chaining.

Forward Chaining Forward chaining describes a chaining procedure in which steps to a complex skill are taught in the order in which they occur in the actual behavioral sequence. Using this type of chaining, the first step in the behavioral chain would initially be taught and successful completion would result in reinforcement. Following acquisition of the initial step, the second step in the chain would be taught and reinforcement provided only for accurate completion of steps one and two. This process would continue until the learner was able to demonstrate all steps independently and accurately. Forward chaining could be implemented to teach the skill steps to any multistep social behavior, such as initiating interactions, leaving interactions, or requesting assistance. In order to do so, a practitioner would develop a task analysis for skill demonstration, ensuring that the task analysis is sufficiently comprehensive to describe complete demonstration of the behavior chain. Skill steps would then be taught in sequence, beginning with the first skill. While the first step is being taught and reinforced, the clinician would assist the learner in completing subsequent steps in the behavior chain. As the learner demonstrates mastery of the initial social skill step, the practitioner would introduce and reinforce the remaining social skill steps in the manner in which they naturally occur until the behavior chain can be completed independently.

DeQuinzio et al. (2008) provide an example of forward chaining applied to social skills teaching. In this study, four children with ASD were taught multistep sharing responses using forward chaining and contingent social interaction. As part of the intervention, study participants were taught to get a toy off a shelf, recruit the attention of another individual, invite the individual to engage in joint play, and engage in a play interaction. Steps to the multistep sharing response were taught across multiple phases, with steps being taught individually and sequentially and reinforcement being provided contingent upon demonstrating the target steps taught within each phase. Results of the study indicated that the forward chaining procedure resulted in an increase in demonstration of the chain of sharing responses across all participants, with all four participants demonstrating 100% of skill steps at the conclusion of the intervention. In another example, Daneshvar et al. (2019) used forward chaining to teach social skills to four children with ASD. Forward chaining was used to teach target social skills, with intervention consisting of introducing a photo of a skill step and the interventionist prompting the participant to demonstrate the step. Additional skill steps were introduced in a similar step in a sequential manner once previous steps were mastered. Further, the forward chaining procedure was compared to a social story intervention used to teach the same skills. Results of the study found that the chaining procedure was effective in rapidly increasing the number of skill steps demonstrated, whereas the social story intervention resulted in minimal change in participant social skill use.

Backward Chaining Backward chaining describes a changing procedure in which a multistep skill is task analyzed and steps are taught in the reverse order from which they naturally occur in the behavior chain. In this manner, individuals are initially taught the final step in the behavior change. Once mastered, the second to last step would be introduced—with intervention proceeding in this manner until all steps to the skill are mastered. Applying backward chaining to social skills teaching is similar to forward chaining, with the only difference being the order in which skill steps are taught and reinforced. Thus, intervention would begin with the development of a comprehensive task analysis of the target social skill. The interventionist would then teach and reinforce the last step in the behavior chain, introducing preceding steps once the learner demonstrates mastery of the social skill steps. Compared to forward chaining, backward chaining has the relative benefit of ensuring that individuals contact the terminal, natural social reinforcer for the behavior chain during each learning trial. Despite this, researchers have found that forward chaining and backward chaining are similar in overall efficacy (e.g., Slocum & Tiger, 2011). As such, it is recommended that client preference be considered in selecting between the chaining procedures (Seaver & Bourret, 2014).

Segal (2016) provides an example of the use of backward chaining within social skills teaching for a 5-year-old individual with ASD. As part of the intervention, backward chaining was utilized to teach skills associated with maintaining back-and-forth interaction. As such, the final step of the chain, identified as asking "how are you," was initially taught and reinforced. Once mastered, the verbalization "good, how are you" was taught and reinforced—with the goal of teaching the sequence of initially saying "hi" to a therapist, followed by "good, how are you?" Results of the study found the intervention to result in an increase in interaction with others and use of target skill steps by the participant. In another study evaluating the effect of backward chaining, McDonnell and Laughlin (1989) taught purchasing skills to four adults with severe disabilities. Within the study, skills for purchasing items at the supermarket and a fast-food restaurant were task analyzed. Using backward chaining, skill steps were taught beginning with the final step. New steps were introduced in a reverse order once participants demonstrated two correct trials without interventionist assistance until all steps in the behavior chain had been taught and were able to be completed independently. All participants in the study improved the accuracy of behavior chain completion following implementation of backward chaining, although one participant failed to demonstrate mastery of the complete behavior chain.

Total-Task Chaining Total-task chaining describes a variation of forward chaining in which instruction and reinforcement is provided for each step in a behavior chain during each session. For skill steps that a learner is unable to complete independently, a clinician would provide guidance in completing. Training would continue in this manner until the learner is able to perform all steps in the behavior chain independently and in their correct sequence. As such, total-task chaining is similar to forward chaining in that a behavior chain is learned and reinforced in the order in which it occurs in real-world settings. However, total-task chaining differs from both forward and backward chaining in that training does not focus on a single step at a time, only progressing to teach and reinforce new steps once mastery of previous steps is indicated. As such, it is possible that total-task chaining results in mastery of skill steps is demonstrated in a non-sequential manner.

Again, implementation of total-task chaining for social skills teaching begins with development of a comprehensive task analysis of the target social skill. The clinician would then present the learner with a cue for skill use. The learner would demonstrate any known skill steps correctly, with the clinician providing guidance in unknown or unmastered skill steps in a sequential manner—allowing for completion of the entire behavior chain. Thus, as with backward chaining, the learner contacts the terminal social reinforcer with each trial of the social sequence. The clinician would continue to provide cues for use of the social skill until the learner is able to demonstrate all steps to the social skill accurately and independently. As with findings of similar efficacy of forward and backward chaining, total-task chaining has been found to be similarly efficacious to other chaining procedures (Kazdin, 2001). Thus, learner preference and data regarding skill acquisition should be considered when identifying a chaining procedure to be implemented.

Several researchers have investigated the utility of total-task chaining for the acquisition of social skills. Genc-Tosun and Kurt (2017) utilized total-task chaining as part of an intervention to teach three learners with ASD to use a speech-generating device to request items. A six-step task analysis was identified for requesting via a speech-generating device. Total-task chaining was used to teach the target behavior, and was combined with either a 0-s or 5-s delay in prompting skill steps. Results indicated that the procedures were effective for all participants in promoting acquisition of the requesting skill, with skill accuracy being maintained up to 12 weeks following termination of intervention procedures. In another study, Gilder (2020) used total-task chaining to teach texting to five children and adolescents with ASD. Learners were instructed to send a text to their friend, with researchers providing support during each step that a learner was unable to demonstrate independently. Participants were considered to have mastered the skill once they were able to complete all steps independently. Results of the study found that total-task chaining was effective in promoting acquisition of skill steps, although additional training was required to improve the content quality of texts sent. It was also noted that intervention effects were maintained at a 1-month follow-up, and that intervention steps generalized to novel persons.

Practical Case Example

Yuki is a 15-year-old child with a diagnosis of ASD who is being seen in a community-based clinic for social skills support. Yuki has expressed feeling isolated from peers and a desire to improve friendships at school and in the community. In collaboration with Yuki and their caregivers, appropriately joining peers in unstructured activities was identified as an intervention target. Yuki's therapist believes that chaining would be effective for teaching the multistep skill.

To develop the intervention, Yuki's therapist initially developed a task analysis of steps to joining in an unstructured activity: demonstrate appropriate physical proximity, get the peers attention, ask to join the activity, and, dependent upon the peer's response, join the activity or find a different activity. Upon reviewing the developed task steps in relation to Yuki's social skills, the therapist decides that total-task chaining would be an appropriate chaining procedure. More specifically, Yuki already possesses some of the skill steps needed to complete the behavior chain and quickly acquires skills through observation and imitation. As such, it was hypothesized that total-task chaining would be an efficient and effective means of teaching the behavior chain.

To begin intervention, the therapist tells Yuki that they will do several role-plays in which the behavior chain can be used. The therapist then engages in a variety of activities (e.g., showing videos to an imaginary peer) and tells Yuki to practice joining in. During the trial, the therapist allows Yuki to demonstrate steps independently. Instruction and prompting is provided when Yuki is unable to demonstrate steps within the behavior chain. Yuki is provided with opportunities to practice the skill until 100% of skill steps are demonstrated independently. At this point, the therapist observes Yuki practice the behavior chain with their caregiver. Similarly, support is provided when Yuki is unable to demonstrate a skill step independently. This practice continues until Yuki is able to demonstrate 100% of skill steps independently with their caregiver.

As Yuki has been observed to be able to perform all skill steps independently in a training setting, the therapist instructs Yuki to use the skill in generalized contexts (e.g., home, community, school). The therapist asks Yuki to identify times at which they may use the skill across contexts, and Yuki reports transitions between classes and after school as points during which joining in unstructured groups would be beneficial. The therapist sets a goal with Yuki to practice the skill at least three times per day and record their success. The following week, Yuki meets with the therapist and indicates that they were successful in using the skill across contexts. Yuki reports that they believe the quality of friendships was improved due to increased interaction with peers. Given that Yuki reported success in using the skill in novel contexts, the therapist determines that no additional use of total-task training for joining in unstructured activities is needed at the current time.

Group Contingencies

Group contingencies seek to modify the behavior of a group of learners by using operant conditioning to apply a single contingency of reinforcement to the behavior of two or more individuals (Cooper, Heron, & Heward, 2020). For example, to increase social interaction in a group setting you might tell a group of eight learners that you're going to be observing how many questions they ask of each other over the next 15 min and if it is ten or more they all get a prize. These types of arrangements have been shown to be extremely effective in promoting a wide range of target behaviors, including social behavior. In fact, group contingencies have been shown to foster positive relationships and improve learners' social status through their implementation, making them ideal for targeting learners' social behavior

(Collins et al., 2019). The exact nature of the contingency determines which subtype of group contingency is being applied and there are three different conceptualizations: interdependent, dependent, and independent.

Interdependent Interdependent group contingencies stipulate a reinforcement contingency to which any member of the group can contribute toward its satisfaction. For example, an interdependent group contingency to increase social interaction might require a group of learners to collectively engage in ten total minutes of social interaction during a 30 min session. The example in the preceding paragraph is another example of an interdependent group contingency. Interdependent group contingencies do not always specify who in the group must exhibit the target behavior; however, they do specify the amount of behavior that needs to be changed. For this reason, some have expressed concern that they may lead to social loafing, whereby one or more members of the group do not engage in the target behavior yet still reap the benefits of the reinforcement contingencies due to the efforts of their peers. Despite this, interdependent group contingencies are the most popular of the three subtypes (Maggin et al., 2012).

Kohler et al. (1995) implemented an interdependent group contingency in a classroom setting of three preschoolers with ASD and their six typically developing peers. All nine students were provided with "Happy Face Charts" that contained empty squares. Each day during a play activity period, the students were instructed that if they all filled the squares on their "Happy Face Charts," they would all get a prize. Otherwise, no one would get a prize. Students could fill squares by organizing play, sharing, and providing assistance to peers. The classroom teachers were responsible for managing the charts and were also allowed to provide any number of prompts to students to engage in the target behaviors throughout the play activity period. Kohler et al. (1995) found that the interdependent contingency drastically increased the students' social interactions during the play activity period.

Dependent Dependent group contingencies arrange a contingency whereby a subset of group members alone are responsible for whether the reinforcement contingency is satisfied. For example, a dependent group contingency for social interaction might require two members of the eight person group to exhibit the 10 min of social interaction necessary for reinforcement after the 30 min session. If these two members together engage in 10 min of social interaction (either with themselves or others), everyone in the group receives reinforcement. If these two members do not engage in 10 min of social interaction, no one receives reinforcement. For this reason, it is often assumed that dependent group contingencies might lead to social pressure or inappropriate social behavior if the dependent members do not satisfy the criterion for reinforcement. Researchers have navigated this issue by keeping the targeted group member or group members a secret so that no one, not even the targeted member, knows who is responsible for satisfying the contingency until after the contingency period has ended and only then if they were successful (e.g., Pasqua et al., 2021).

Although there are numerous examples of dependent group contingencies in the literature, there are no clear examples supporting their use to promote social skill use in individuals with ASD. One study examined their use to promote appropriate social behavior in a self-contained special education middle school classroom. Each day, Hansen and Lignugaris-Kraft (2005) randomly selected two students from the eight student classroom but did not reveal them. These students had to exhibit four positive statements toward peers during a 15-min activity period. If they were able to do so, all eight students could select a reward from a prize box at the end of the school day. The data demonstrate a clear increase in peer-directed positive statements under the effect of the dependent group contingency over baseline levels. Because students never knew if they were the target student, relatively stable increases were observed throughout the duration of the study as all students believed they might have been selected that day. Hansen and Lignugaris-Kraft (2005) demonstrated continued effectiveness of this strategy even in the face of a fading phase which involved a thinner and more variable schedule of reinforcement through the use of dice rolling.

Independent Independent group contingencies describe a type of contingency in which reinforcement is provided to members of a group based on their own performance against some criterion. As such, individual group contingencies can be thought of as "every individual for themselves," as the performance of one individual in the group in no way impacts the eligibility for reinforcement of other individuals within the group. Using the previous requirement of 10 min of social interaction during a 30-min session, an independent group contingency would provide a reward only to those group members that meet or exceed this criterion. Thus, if one group member only interacts with peers for 5 min, they would not be eligible for reinforcement. Independent group contingencies eliminate any potential social loafing within the group, but may decrease the likelihood that group members provide positive peer pressure to others in the group through encouraging skill use.

Independent group contingencies have been frequently evaluated in the intervention literature and found to improve a range of outcomes (e.g., Little et al., 2015). However, independent group contingencies have rarely been applied to social skills teaching for individuals with ASD. In one of the only extant examples, Pokorski et al. (2019) implemented an independent group contingency with preschool-age students with multiple or severe disabilities. One of the students included in the study was reported to have a diagnosis of ASD. Within the study, each student contacted reinforcement for demonstrating "good friend" behaviors. Once students had been observed to demonstrate five "good friend" behaviors, they were eligible for reinforcement. Results of the study demonstrate that the independent group contingency was effective in increasing the frequency of appropriate social interactions for five of six students.

Case Example A school psychologist teaches a weekly social skills group with five students with ASD. The therapist provides instruction in target social skills using a manualized curriculum. Although participants demonstrate the ability to use the target social skills within the social skills group setting, teachers report that group participants do not use target social skills in the classroom. As such, the school psychologist decides to implement a group contingency to promote social skill use in non-training settings.

The school psychologist decides to set up an independent group contingency, in which reinforcement is provided to each group participant for demonstrating five instances of target social skill use within the classroom. Teachers are provided data sheets which identify the target social skill and provide space for tracking the observed frequency of skill use. Next, the school psychologist meets with group participants to explain the group contingency. Participants are informed that they will be able to select from a menu of preferred items for using the target social skill within the classroom. Participants are told that their teachers will be recording instances of skill use and sending daily reports of skill use to the school psychologist, and that for each day that they demonstrate the target skill a minimum of five times, they will be able to select a preferred reinforcer.

After explaining intervention procedures to group members, teachers begin to record instances of social skill use in the classroom. At the end of each day, teachers provide the school psychologist with the frequency of skill use. Each group member who demonstrated skill use at least five times within the classroom is then allowed to select a reinforcer. After 1 week of implementation, the school psychologist observes that teacher reports of skill use have increased for all group members. Anecdotal teacher reports also reveal that participants demonstrate higher rates of target social skill use within the classroom. Given the efficacy of the intervention, the school psychologist continues to implement the intervention, regularly changing the skill monitored by teachers to match the skill taught in group.

Conclusion

The field of behavior analysis has produced several intervention technologies that have found to be effective in teaching and maintaining appropriate social skill use in individuals with ASD. Differential reinforcement, chaining, and group contingencies have each been identified as effective for this purpose and have considerable evidence to support them as such. Differential reinforcement is ideal for addressing performance deficits, particularly when challenging behavior or inappropriate social behavior is present. Chaining is useful for addressing acquisition deficits where it can be used to teach more complex multistep social skills through task analyses. Group contingencies are valued for their innate social nature and efficiency in modifying the social behavior of groups of learners. Practitioners are encouraged to consider these behavior analytic techniques as stand-alone interventions or as components of larger intervention packages.

References

Axelrod, S., McElrath, K. K., & Wine, B. (2012). Applied behavior analysis: Autism and beyond. *Behavioral Interventions, 27*, 1–15.

Baer, D. M., Wolf, M. M., & Risley, T. R. (1968). Some current dimensions of applied behavior analysis. *Journal of Applied Behavior Analysis, 1*, 91–97.

Baer, D. M., Wolf, M. M., & Risley, T. R. (1987). Some still-current dimensions of applied behavior analysis. *Journal of Applied Behavior Analysis, 20*, 313–327.

Call, N. A., Pabico, R. S., Findley, A. J., & Valentino, A. L. (2011). Differential reinforcement with and without blocking as treatment for elopement. *Journal of Applied Behavior Analysis, 44*, 903–907.

Cooper, J. O., Heron, T. E., & Heward, W. L. (2020). *Applied behavior analysis*. Pearson.

Collins, T. A., Hawkins, R. O., Heidelburg, K., & Hill, K. (2019). Group contingencies. In K. C. Radley & E. H. Dart (Eds.), *Handbook of behavioral interventions in schools: Multi-tiered systems of support* (pp. 204–233). Oxford University Press.

Daneshvar, S. D., Charlop, M. H., & Berry Malmberg, D. (2019). A treatment comparison study of a photo activity schedule and social stories for teaching social skills to children with Autism Spectrum Disorder: Brief report. *Developmental Neurorehabilitation, 22*, 209–214.

DeQuinzio, J. A., Townsend, D. B., & Poulson, C. L. (2008). The effects of forward chaining and contingent social interaction on the acquisition of complex sharing responses by children with autism. *Research in Autism Spectrum Disorders, 2*, 264–275.

Fantino, E., & Logan, C. A. (1979). *The experimental analysis of behavior: A biological perspective*. Freeman.

Foxall, G. R. (2010). Invitation to consumer behavior analysis. *Journal of Organizational Behavior Management, 30*, 92–109.

Gadaire, D. M., Marshall, G., & Brissett, E. (2017). Differential reinforcement of low rate responding in social skills training. *Learning and Motivation, 60*, 34–40.

Genc-Tosun, D., & Kurt, O. (2017). Teaching multi-step requesting to children with autism spectrum disorder using systematic instruction and a speech-generating device. *Augmentative and Alternative Communication, 33*, 213–223.

Gilder, J. (2020). *Teaching texting on a smartphone to children and adolescents with Autism Spectrum Disorder (ASD)*. Doctoral dissertation, The Claremont Graduate University.

Hansen, S. D., & Lignugaris-Kraft, B. (2005). Effects of a dependent group contingency on the verbal interactions of middle school students with emotional disturbance. *Behavioral Disorders, 30*, 170–184.

Johnson, K. A., Vladescu, J. C., Kodak, T., & Sidener, T. M. (2017). An assessment of differential reinforcement procedures for learners with autism spectrum disorder. *Journal of Applied Behavior Analysis, 50*, 290–303.

Kazdin, A. E. (2001). *Behavior modification in applied settings* (6th ed.). Thomson Learning.

Kohler, F. W., Strain, P. S., Hoyson, M., Davis, L., Donina, W. M., & Rapp, N. (1995). Using a group-oriented contingency to increase social interactions between children with autism and their peers: A preliminary analysis of corollary supportive behaviors. *Behavior Modification, 19*, 10–32.

Konczak, L. J., & Johnson, C. M. (1983). Reducing inappropriate verbalizations in a sheltered workshop through differential reinforcement of other behavior. *Education and Training of the Mentally Retarded, 18*, 120–124.

Lehman, P. K., & Geller, E. S. (2004). Behavior analysis and environmental protection: Accomplishments and potential for more. *Behavior and Social Issues, 13*, 13–33.

Little, S. G., Akin-Little, A., & O'Neill, K. (2015). Group contingency interventions with children—1980–2010: A meta-analysis. *Behavior Modification, 39*(2), 322–341.

MacNaul, H. L., & Neely, L. C. (2018). Systematic review of differential reinforcement of alternative behavior without extinction for individuals with autism. *Behavior Modification, 42*, 398–421.

Maggin, D. M., Johnson, A. H., Chafouleas, S. M., Ruberto, L. M., & Berggren, M. (2012). A systematic evidence review of school-based group contingency interventions for students with challenging behavior. *Journal of School Psychology, 50*, 625–654.
McDonnell, J., & Laughlin, B. (1989). A comparison of backward and concurrent chaining strategies in teaching community skills. *Education and Training in Mental Retardation, 24*, 230–238.
Pasqua, J. L., Dufrene, B. A., LaBrot, Z. C., Radley, K., Dart, E. H., & Lown, E. (2021). Evaluating the independent group contingency: "Mystery Student" on improving behaviors in head start classrooms. *Psychology in the Schools, 58*, 1361–1379.
Pokorski, E. A., Barton, E. E., & Ledford, J. R. (2019). Assessing the differential effects of known and mystery rewards in a preschool-based group contingency. *Journal of Early Intervention, 41*, 256–275.
Repp, A. C., Klett, S. Z., Sosebee, L. H., & Speir, N. C. (1975). Differential effects of four token conditions on rate and choice of responding in a matching-to-sample task. *American Journal of Mental Deficiency, 80*, 51–56.
Seaver, J. L., & Bourret, J. C. (2014). An evaluation of response prompts for teaching behavior chains. *Journal of Applied Behavior Analysis, 47*, 777–792.
Segal, E. A. (2016). *Initiating conversation by a kindergarten-aged child with autism spectrum disorder*. Unpublished senior thesis, James Madison University.
Skinner, B. F. (1966). What is the experimental analysis of behavior? *Journal of the Experimental Analysis of Behavior, 9*, 213–218.
Skinner, B. F. (1971). Operant conditioning. *The Encyclopedia of Education, 7*, 29–33.
Slocum, S. K., & Tiger, J. H. (2011). An assessment of the efficiency of and child preference for forward and backward chaining. *Journal of Applied Behavior Analysis, 44*, 793–805.
Weston, R., Hodges, A. & Davis, T. N. (2018). Differential Reinforcement of Other Behaviors to Treat Challenging Behaviors Among Children With Autism: A Systematic and Quality Review. *Behavior Modification, 42*, 584–609.
Winett, R. A., Moore, J. F., & Anderson, E. S. (1991). Extending the concept of social validity: Behavior analysis for disease prevention and health promotion. *Journal of Applied Behavior Analysis, 24*, 215–230.

Chapter 12
Practical Considerations

The previous chapters have highlighted a variety of social skills teaching strategies that have empirical support as useful and effective in promoting social skill acquisition and broader social skill competency. Despite the utility of the strategies described in previous chapters, many researchers have pointed to findings suggesting only modest overall effects of social skills teaching (e.g., Bellini & Akullian, 2007). This has led to some suggesting that social skills teaching be rethought entirely (e.g., Gresham, 1998). Factors that have limited the confidence that some have in the general utility of social skills teaching are described below, as well as potential considerations and future directions that may strengthen the empirical support of social skills teaching as a broad class of intervention.

Generalization

Bellini and Akullian (2007) highlighted one of the primary limitations of social skills training—generalization of learned skills across persons, places, and other stimuli. Bellini and colleagues' meta-analysis highlighted that social skills teaching strategies are often effective in promoting behavior change within the teaching setting; however, generalized effects of social skills training were typically more attenuated. Similar findings of limited generalized effects have been found in other studies (e.g., Hutchins et al., 2020; Whalon et al., 2015). Thus, given that some procedures discussed in previous chapters have suggested greater generalized effects than that observed in meta-analyses of broader social skills teaching interventions, it would behoove researchers and practitioners to devote particular attention to those interventions and studies in which stronger generalization effects have been demonstrated.

K. C Radley, E. H. Dart, *Social Skills Teaching for Individuals with Autism*,
Springer Series on Child and Family Studies,
https://doi.org/10.1007/978-3-030-91665-7_12

Although many researchers have noted the lack of generalized effects of social skills teaching interventions, equally problematic is that many social skills teaching intervention studies have not assessed for generalization of effects. For example, the meta-analysis conducted by Hutchins et al. (2020) found that only 3 of the 25 identified studies assessed for generalization—fewer studies than the already low rate of generalization data collection documented by Bellini and Akullian (2007). The lack of assessment of generalized effects of social skills teaching, coupled with the limited generalized effects observed in those studies that have assessed generalization, further emphasizes the need for rigorous and comprehensive evaluation of social skills teaching strategies. Again, consumers of research and intervention materials are encouraged to carefully consider the empirical support for teaching strategies selected for use—with a particular emphasis on evidence for generalized skill use.

Given the noted limitations with respect to generalization of social skills teaching, researchers and practitioners should also endeavor to incorporate generalization-promoting technologies in social skills teaching whenever possible. In describing strategies that may promote generalized responding, Stokes and Osnes (1989) identified contacting natural consequences, reinforcing occurrences of generalization, training sufficient stimulus and response exemplars, incorporating common physical and social stimuli, and incorporating self-mediated stimuli as some means of augmenting the generalized effects of interventions. Applied to social skills, these strategies may consist of teaching social skills in context—not in contrived settings, but in naturalistic settings and with peers with whom individuals may naturally use newly learned skills. Doing so also allows individuals to contact natural sources of reinforcement (e.g., peer responses) that may maintain skill use in the absence of contrived reinforcers for demonstrating target social skills. Ultimately, the goal of social skills teaching is not skill use in decontextualized pull-out settings, but that skills taught allow greater access to and inclusion in naturalistic settings—thus, incorporating strategies such as those identified by Stokes and Osnes are central to the overarching goals of social skills teaching.

Maintenance

Maintenance of social skills refers to the durability of behavior change following social skills teaching. Similar to generalization, several researchers have noted that the maintained effects of social skills teaching are lesser than those observed during training conditions (e.g., Hutchins et al., 2020; Bellini & Akullian, 2007). Maintenance of skills should be proactively addressed, with planning for maintenance of skills being incorporated to all social skills teaching interventions.

As with generalization, researchers have sought to identify strategies that increase the likelihood that a skill will be maintained over time. Maintenance of skills may be proactively addressed through teaching in context and allowing for naturalistic reinforcers to be contacted following skill use. Additionally, social skills teaching strategies should incorporate regular checks for maintenance of previously learned skills. Often, social skills teaching progresses in a sequential manner with teaching only addressing the current skill. Instead, social skills teaching should revisit previously taught skills to ensure skill maintenance—providing reteaching when maintenance is not observed. Similarly, maintenance may be promoted by ensuring that reinforcement is contacted not only for the skill currently being taught, but also for previously taught skills. Using this strategy, those conducting social skills teaching may ensure that recipients of social skills teaching do not experience ratio strain, or a stoppage of responding when a schedule of reinforcement is thinned too quickly.

Narrow Focus

In addition to concerns related to the generalizability and maintained effects of social skills teaching, social skills teaching has been critiqued as focusing too narrowly on pre-defined social behaviors. Indeed, some social skills teaching interventions may rigidly teach steps to social skill use—providing teaching in only one way of using a particular social skill. Teaching in this manner may result in development of a narrow repertoire of social skills, or skills that are decontextualized from the setting in which they occur.

One potential strategy for addressing this limitation of social skills training is through incorporation of lag schedules of reinforcement. Lag schedules of reinforcement describe procedures in which reinforcement is provided not based on accuracy of skill use, but on a response being topographically different from one or more prior responses (Page & Neuringer, 1985). To provide an example, a lag 2 schedule would require a response to be topographically different from the preceding two responses in order to access reinforcement.

Although a relatively novel intervention procedure, lag schedules of reinforcement have garnered support as a useful means for promoting accurate skill use while augmenting the behavioral repertoire of individuals in both training and generalization settings. In an early example, Lee et al. (2002) found lag schedules to increase variability in responding to social questions of participants with ASD. Radley et al. (2019) found lag schedules to result in increased variability in responding to nonparticipant peers. Finally, in a systematic review of lag schedule, Silbaugh et al. (2021) opined that lag schedules represented a promising intervention strategy for individuals with ASD. Taken together, the empirical support for lag schedules suggests that they may be a useful means of addressing challenges related to the narrow focus of social skills teaching. Although further research is necessary, lag schedules of reinforcement hold potential in supporting social skill use that is adaptive to contextual features of a social setting—allowing social skill use to be more natural and responsive to unique environmental demands.

Identification of Skills to Target

As discussed previously (see Chap. 2), it is necessary to determine which social skills will be taught or reinforced before any work can begin. This can be accomplished through a variety of methods. Perhaps the most common are the manualized intervention packages that provide practitioners with a scope and sequence of social behaviors deemed suitable for teaching (e.g., Social Skills Improvement System; Gresham & Elliott, 2008); however, other options include checklists and rating scales such as the Autism Social Skills Profile (ASSP: Bellini, 2006) or the School Social Behavior Scales (SSBS; Merrell, 2008). Finally, practitioners may also rely on interviews with clients, caregivers, and other stakeholders (e.g., teachers, employers) and direct observation of clients or others in relevant environments to inform the selection of target skills. Each method of social skill selection has benefits and drawbacks. For example, manualized curricula provide a full list of skills and materials to teach them and often have a rating scale or other assessment that can be used to identify which skills should be prioritized. On the other hand, manualized curricula are restricted in their range and may not be appropriate for all clients. Additionally, social behavior is very nuanced and what is considered appropriate may change across settings, people, or time. Thus, we support an individualized social skill curriculum plan for each client that incorporates their unique needs and desires related to their social functioning. To highlight this point, we will use the variable of setting to demonstrate how a one-size-fits-all approach may not be effective.

Setting Specific Social Skills

Individuals are expected to function across many different environments including home, their community, school or other educational settings, and a workplace. Across these environments, individuals often have to adapt to the behavioral and social expectations that are present. Some expectations, like those in a school building, are developed and enforced by a few individuals (e.g., teacher, administrator, school district personnel) without much input from the majority (i.e., the students). Other settings may function similarly (e.g., an authoritative household) or differently (e.g., a more democratic household). Finally, the expectations in some settings are developed by those currently occupying the space at that moment (e.g., a playground, a park). For example, a group of adults holding a meditation group in a small park may expect others entering the park to respect the calm and quiet environment they have created. On the other hand, a group of teenagers in the same park after dark may be acting under an entirely different set of social expectations. The point being that there is no set of social behaviors or responses that will be universally appropriate in a given time and place.

When developing a social skills treatment program for a client, it is crucial to consider these factors to determine which skills will result in the most therapeutic benefit. This will require incorporating the perspectives of various individuals, including the client and other stakeholders, to ensure that the behaviors being taught and reinforced are relevant. Murray and Doren (2013) provided an example of how this process might look for a vocational setting. Using the Working at Gaining Employment Skills (WAGES) curriculum and incorporating input from the clients and their teachers, Murray and Doren demonstrated a large increase in occupational skills related to vocational success but fewer effects for other social skills such as cooperation, self-control, and assertion. These data highlight the restricted range of manualized curricula but also emphasize their effectiveness when used for a particular purpose. A meta-analysis by Park et al. (2016) supported the general effectiveness of social skills training specific to vocational settings and found these programs to confer moderate gains within this domain of social functioning ($d = 0.56$).

Social Skills and Autism

Related to issues of individualization and client benefit is the recent increase in communication from individuals in and adjacent to the Autism community about the appropriateness (or lack thereof) of teaching social skills to neurodiverse individuals. Although many individuals may be the recipient of intervention services targeting social behavior, individuals with autism are more likely to receive these services than others due to social and communication deficits being a defining feature of the condition. A recent commentary by Bottema-Beutel et al. (2018) provides a comprehensive analysis of the state of the social skill teaching literature for individuals with autism as well as possible explanations for why current social skills teaching techniques are inadequate. They distinguish between "top down" and "bottom up" social rules or norms. Top down rules "consist of culturally specific expectations and frames of reference that allow interaction partners to ascribe social actions to their interaction partner's utterances…" (p. 955). On the other hand, bottom up social processing involves "negotiating and reconfiguring social norms within interactions" (p. 955).

It is the latter that they assert are potentially harmed by overly stringent social skills teaching as individuals are deprived of the opportunity to engage in bottom up social processing in favor of routinized social interactions instilled by manualized curricula. They conclude by offering three recommendations to the field: (1) Incorporate conversation analysis and literature from sociolinguistics to determine which skills should be taught and how; (2) move from a framework of teaching normative social behaviors to one where we instead teach the skills necessary to make sense of pragmatic language and other process-oriented approaches; and (3) develop training programs targeting neurotypical individuals aimed at eliminating stereotypes of individuals with autism. The ideas and recommendations described in this article are extremely useful and can be incorporated into the strategies that have been described in the earlier chapters of this book. It is important for clinicians to work together with their clients and any relevant stakeholders (e.g., caregivers, partners) to determine whether there is a clear need to intervene in the area of social behavior. Keep in mind that interventions to address acquisition deficits (i.e., skill deficits) appear very different than those that are aimed at addressing performance deficits and that the former may be more controversial than the latter as the teaching is focused on how rather than how much or when. Regardless, all social behavioral targets and goals based upon them will be made in relation to whatever social norms and conventions exist in a particular setting or for a certain behavior. The decision to intervene in this area must be made with care and with the client's best interest in mind rather than others' (e.g., classroom teachers, caregivers).

Conclusion

In conclusion, applying one or more of the many social skills intervention strategies described in this book requires careful consideration of the practical issues described in this last chapter. Programming for generalization, maintenance, and variability in skill exhibition is important for client independence and continued success. Further, becoming flexible about which skills are taught and how they are taught is important when considering client autonomy and respecting their diverse needs. Allowing clients to express themselves authentically rather than engaging in rigid and mechanical social interactions can only be accomplished if the methods we are using to teach social behavior are themselves not rigid and mechanical. Collecting input from clients and other relevant stakeholders can increase the likelihood that our social skills teaching frameworks are most supportive of our clients' needs.

References

Bellini, S. (2006). *Autism social skills profile*. AAPC Publishing.

Bellini, S., & Akullian, J. (2007). A meta-analysis of video modeling and video self-modeling interventions for children and adolescents with autism spectrum disorders. *Exceptional Children, 73*, 264–287.

Bottema-Beutel, K., Park, H., & Kim, S. Y. (2018). Commentary on social skills training curricula for individuals with ASD: Social interaction, authenticity, and stigma. *Journal of Autism and Developmental Disorders, 48*, 953–964.

Gresham, F. M. (1998). Social skills training: Should we raze, remodel, or rebuild? *Behavioral Disorders, 24*, 19–25.

Gresham, F. M., & Elliott, S. N. (2008). *Social skills improvement system. Rating scales manual.* Pearson.

Hutchins, N. S., Burke, M. D., Bowman-Perrott, L., Tarlow, K. R., & Hatton, H. (2020). The effects of social skills interventions for students with EBD and ASD: A single-case meta-analysis. *Behavior Modification, 44*, 773–794.

Lee, R., McComas, J. J., & Jawor, J. (2002). The effects of differential and lag reinforcement schedules on varied verbal responding by individuals with autism. *Journal of Applied Behavior Analysis, 35*, 391–402.

Merrell, K. W. (2008). *School social behavior scales user's guide* (2nd ed.). Brookes Publishing.

Murray, C., & Doren, B. (2013). The effects of working at gaining employment skills on the social and vocational skills of adolescents with disabilities: A school-based intervention. *Rehabilitation Counseling Bulletin, 56*, 96–107.

Page, S., & Neuringer, A. (1985). Variability is an operant. *Journal of Experimental Psychology: Animal Behavior Processes, 11*, 429–452.

Park, E. Y., Kim, J., & Kim, S. S. (2016). Meta-analysis of the effect of job-related social skill training for secondary students with disabilities. *Journal of Vocational Rehabilitation, 44*, 123–133.

Radley, K. C., Dart, E. H., Helbig, K. A., Schrieber, S. R., & Ware, M. E. (2019). An evaluation of the additive effects of lag schedules of reinforcement. *Developmental Neurorehabilitation, 22*, 180–191.

Silbaugh, B. C., Murray, C., Kelly, M. P., & Healy, O. (2021). A systematic synthesis of lag schedule research in individuals with autism and other populations. *Review Journal of Autism and Developmental Disorders, 8*, 92–107.

Stokes, T. F., & Osnes, P. G. (1989). An operant pursuit of generalization. *Behavior Therapy, 20*, 337–355.

Whalon, K. J., Conroy, M. A., Martinez, J. R., & Werch, B. L. (2015). School-based peer-related social competence interventions for children with autism spectrum disorder: A meta-analysis and descriptive review of single case research design studies. *Journal of Autism and Developmental Disorders, 45*, 1513–1531.

Index

K. C Radley, E. H. Dart, *Social Skills Teaching for Individuals with Autism*,
Springer Series on Child and Family Studies,
https://doi.org/10.1007/978-3-030-91665-7

T

The manufacturer's authorised representative in the EU is Springer Nature Customer Service Centre GmbH, Europaplatz 3, 69115 Heidelberg, Germany. If you have any concerns regarding our products, please contact ProductSafety@springernature.com

Printed and bound by CPI Group (UK) Ltd, Croydon, CR0 4YY
30/09/2026
02225470-0014